Caring for People
with Alzheimer's Disease

Endings

by Lynn Kozma,
a retired registered nurse who served
in the Army Nurse Corps, Air Forces, in World War II

Frail as porcelain
she sits, unmoving
except for bone-thin hands
mending with care
forgotten clothes
which are not there—
threading unseen needles,
moistening fingertips
from parchment lips,
knotting the thread
carefully.

There—one more finished—
smoothing the wrinkles away,
softly laying it by,
slipping back
to the early May
of her life
as easily as breathing.

My planet—earth;
hers—a distant star.
Impossible to travel
that far.

Caring for People with Alzheimer's Disease

A Training Manual for Direct Care Providers

by

Gayle Andresen, R.N.-C., M.S., A.N.P./G.N.P.

in association with

Health Education Development System, Inc.
and Cooperative Health Education Program
(HEDS/CHEP)

Fort Meade, South Dakota

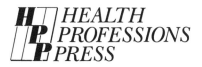

HEALTH
PROFESSIONS
PRESS

Baltimore • London • Toronto • Sydney

Health Professions Press, Inc.
Post Office Box 10624
Baltimore, Maryland 21285-0624

Copyright © 1995 by Health Professions Press.
All rights reserved.

Typeset by Signature Typesetting & Design, Baltimore, Maryland.
Manufactured in the United States of America by
The Maple Press Company, York, Pennsylvania.

Permission to reprint the following poem is gratefully acknowledged:

Endings from Kozma, L. (1987). *When I am an old woman I shall wear purple.*
Watsonville, CA: Papier-Mache Press; reprinted by permission.

Library of Congress Cataloging-in-Publication Data
Andresen, Gayle.
   Caring for people with Alzheimer's disease : a training manual for direct care
   providers / Gayle Andresen ; in association with Health Education Development
   System, Inc./Cooperative Health Education Program (HEDS/CHEP).
      p.   cm.
   Includes bibliographical references and index.
   ISBN 1-878812-22-X
   1. Alzheimer's disease—Patients—Long-term care—Handbooks, manuals, etc.
2. Alzheimer's disease—Patients—Care—Handbooks, manuals, etc.   I. Health
Education Development System, Inc. / Cooperative Health Education Program.
II. Title.
   [DNLM: 1. Alzheimer's Disease—handbooks.   2. Long-Term Care—
methods—handbooks.   WM 34 A561c 1995]
RC523.A53   1995
362.1'96831—dc20
DNLM/DLC
for Library of Congress   94-31057
                                                                           CIP

British Library Cataloguing-in-Publication data are available from the British
Library.

Contents

List of Tables and Figures

Preface

Over 4 million Americans have Alzheimer's disease. This number is an everyday reality for those who either have Alzheimer's disease or care for people with the disease. This manual is for caregivers, whether they are family members or staff members of a health care facility.

The manual is a result of a joint project begun in 1991 to provide training for staff who care for people with Alzheimer's disease in long-term and acute care facilities. The project was initiated by the Health Education Development System, Inc. and Cooperative Health Education Program (HEDS/CHEP) in Fort Meade, South Dakota. Over 60 rural health care facilities in South Dakota, Wyoming, Nebraska, Montana, and North Dakota are members of HEDS/CHEP. Through their cooperation, they bring continuing health education to their staff and communities.

Health care staffs were seeing an increasing number of people with Alzheimer's disease and other dementias, and they talked with HEDS/CHEP about the need for training—not just once a year, but ongoing and frequent training in their facilities. They wanted all staff having any contact with people with Alzheimer's disease to receive training. They wanted training material for teaching their staff. They wanted information on how to present the training. They wanted the material segmented so it could be used for a 1- or 2-hour inservice. They wanted it to be easy to use. *And* they wanted it to include information needed by all levels of staff (e.g., nurses, nursing assistants, social workers, dietitians, housekeepers, activities directors).

It was evident that a professional experienced in geriatric care and teaching was needed. We found such a person in Gayle Andresen, a geriatric nurse practitioner, an instructor of family medicine at the University of Colorado School of Medicine, and a clinician at A.F. Williams Center in Denver, Colorado. We realized the benefit this project could have to health care workers beyond the HEDS/CHEP consortium area. To that end, we invited the participation of two other continuing education agencies in South Dakota: the Lewis & Clark Health Education and Services Agency, with constituents in South Dakota and Nebraska; and the Sioux Falls Area Health Education Center, with constituents in South Dakota and Minnesota. Fortunately, the Bush Foundation of St. Paul, Minnesota, agreed to help support our endeavor.

Fifty-three health care workers—nurses, social workers, activities directors, and nursing assistants—participated in a 2-day "train-the-trainer" workshop presented by Gayle Andresen to "test" the manual for us. During the 2-day session, they learned more about Alzheimer's disease and how to use the manual. When they returned to their communities, they used the manual to teach health care staff and others in the community. Later, they told us what they liked, what they did not like, and what else they wanted.

This manual provides most of the information needed about what Alzheimer's disease is, how to care for the people with the disease, and how to care for yourself. We strongly encourage the "student" and the instructor to draw from other timely sources to supplement their information and learning. The suggested readings in the back of the manual offer an excellent starting point.

Jan Smith, M.S.W.
Health Education Development System, Inc.
and Cooperative Health Education Program

Acknowledgments

We would like to thank Gayle Andresen for taking on this project amidst her already busy schedule and conveying what this is all about—understanding and giving better care to people with Alzheimer's disease; the Bush Foundation for funding the project that made this manual possible; all members of HEDS/CHEP for recognizing the need for this training; the 53 health care professionals who participated in the demonstration project for testing the first draft of the manual and giving us terrific suggestions for improvements; Jan Smith, M.S.W., Vice President and Associate Director of HEDS/CHEP, for researching the need for and spearheading the project that resulted in this manual; Charlotte Forsberg, M.A., retired English professor, for editing the preproduction manual; Lewis & Clark Health Education & Services Agency and Sioux Falls AHEC/CHES for participating in the development and testing of the manual; the Alzheimer's Association, Chicago, Illinois, for giving us excellent references to "persons in the know" as we began this project, helping us locate some of the authors whose material is used in the manual, and allowing us to use some of their articles in the manual; and Lynn Kozma, R.N., Aaron B. Lerner, M.D., Wilson Pace, M.D., Marshall F. Folstein, M.D., Eric Pfieffer, M.D., J.A. Yesavage, M.D., and Plenum Press for allowing us to use their work in this manual.

Health Education Development System, Inc.
and Cooperative Health Education Program

I would like to thank the Alzheimer's Association, Metro Denver Chapter, Denver, Colorado, for the time and effort spent helping me find the best resources; Anne Robinson and colleagues for allowing me to draw from their materials and references; and the special patients with Alzheimer's disease for giving me many helpful and practical ideas about care. They have been extraordinarily patient when I didn't understand their words or gestures. They have taught me to have patience with patients!

Gayle Andresen

Introduction

The purpose of this manual is to improve the level of care provided to people with Alzheimer's disease or related disorders. This can be accomplished by educating those who care for, or come in contact with, people with Alzheimer's disease. The manual is intended for health care professionals—including nurses, nursing assistants, social workers, and dietary workers—and family members who are caregivers at home.

PHILOSOPHY OF THE TRAINING CURRICULUM

Each person is unique, with a lifetime of experiences and memories, and each individual is entitled to live a life of dignity. All people, especially those with dementia, need a sense of trust and control in their environment. Fostering this sense requires that everyone having contact with the person with dementia be knowledgeable, compassionate, and sensitive to the importance of verbal and nonverbal interactions.

USING THE TRAINING MANUAL

The manual is divided into seven units and an Instructor's Guide. The Instructor's Guide provides tips for preparing for a class, teaching a lesson, and using transparencies.

CONTENT OF EACH UNIT

The first six units are designed to be presented within about 50 minutes or less, and correspond with each other. However, individual units can be presented independently, or divided and presented in shorter portions to meet time constraints.

The first six units include learning objectives, lesson content, a quiz, and instructor help.

Learning objectives are stated at the beginning of each unit. The objectives list what is to be taught—or more appropriately, what is to be learned—in each unit.

Education or lesson content provides a structured guide for teaching each unit. Headings are used to identify the major sections of each lesson. Most of the units also include figures and tables, which can be used as supplemental material in teaching the unit.

A *quiz* covering the lesson content is included at the end of each unit. (Answers to the quizzes may be found in Appendix D.) Use of the quizzes is optional; however, they are helpful in measuring instructor effectiveness.

Instructor help provides suggestions to trainers on ways to develop and present the unit, and suggests activities to use during sessions.

Unit 7 provides information on the benefits and basic provisions of special care units in long-term care facilities. Much of the content can be incorporated, when appropriate, into any of the other units.

Appendix A contains five assessment tools used to evaluate dementia. These screening tools can be used by a professional who is well versed in taking medical histories. Instructors may use these tools as teaching aids for any of the units, particularly Unit 1. Appendix B contains teaching supplements that can be used for making transparencies or handouts. Appendix C contains suggested readings. It is divided into two sections, "Resources for Professionals" and "Resources for Families." The first section provides supplemental reading suggestions for the instructor or student for each unit. The second section is for anyone who comes in contact with a person with Alzheimer's disease. It includes topics such as references, diaries, institutional care, activities, children, teenagers, newsletters, and resource centers.

Instructor's Guide

The purpose of the Instructor's Guide is to provide assistance for the instructor or trainer. Tips are offered on how to prepare for an education session and how to conduct a session. These tips include such details as preparing materials and equipment and reading resources prior to the session. Points are provided for using various teaching methods, and suggestions are given for designing and using overhead transparencies. Additionally, the basic principles of how adults learn are presented. These principles can help the instructor decide the methods to use to teach and underscore the importance of openness on the part of the instructor—that is, openness to questions, puzzled looks, or the need for discussion. The role of the instructor is critical in presenting information, stimulating the trainees to learn, and creating an environment in which they can learn.

TIPS FOR GETTING STARTED

Add your own ideas to the presentation. Adding your own ideas will help personalize the material and add to the credibility of the instructor. Illustrate concepts or techniques using your own experiences with people with Alzheimer's disease or call upon trainees to describe their experiences.

Encourage discussion. It is important to involve trainees by asking for their ideas and opinions. Some of the sessions will include specific suggestions for involving trainees, as in role playing or brief, planned presentations. A blackboard, whiteboard, or newsprint pad can be useful for keeping track of important points generated during the discussion.

Use audiovisuals, such as overhead transparencies and videotapes. Transparencies help trainees follow the session. Videotapes are very useful for illustrating some of the behaviors that will be covered in the sessions. *Managing and Understanding Behavior Problems in Alzheimer's Disease and Related Disorders* is a 10-module videotape series developed by Dr. Linda Teri and colleagues from the University of Washington Medical Center. Tapes from the series are referred to in each Unit: Instructor Help. The videotapes may be purchased for $250 from the Northwest Geriatric Education Center, University of Washington, HL-23, Seattle, Washington 98195, (206) 685-7478. The series is geared toward institutional staff, families, and in-home caregivers.

Read some of the resources listed in the Suggested Readings for the unit you are presenting. Reading the resources will give you a greater depth of understanding of the material and will help generate ideas that can be used to enhance your presentation.

Use some or all of the supplemental material in the units. All units except Units 5 and 7 include one or more pages of supplemental material. These materials are for enhancement of the educational presentation and include figures and tables. Use the materials that are relevant for your particular group of trainees or you may wish to design your own.

"Test" the trainees' knowledge. Each unit includes quizzes designed as mastery tests, meaning that the trainee should be expected to answer at least half of the questions correctly. However, please look on the quizzes as learning tools. The important thing is for the trainees to learn.

Be prepared several days before the date of the presentation. Use the following as a checklist to make certain you are ready for the educational presentation:

1. Read *all* the material for the unit you plan to teach.
2. Prepare notes in a way to ensure that you will not forget important material (e.g., 4" × 6" cards—make a separate card for each main point).
3. Prepare transparencies and other teaching aids (e.g., videorecorders, blackboard).
4. Preview all videotapes you plan to use. If you will be using only a segment of a videotape, advance the tape to that segment so that it is ready to show.
5. Copy any handouts you may wish to add to the material in the manual.

6. Bring extra pencils to the classroom—somebody always needs one.

ADULT TEACHING/LEARNING PRINCIPLES

Whether you are an inexperienced teacher or have taught classes before, it might be helpful to review some principles that affect the way adults learn. These principles may be used as a template against which to evaluate plans for teaching any of the sessions. Ask yourself about the relevancy of the information you plan to teach. How can you best stimulate the "need to know" among the trainees? How open are you to the ideas of others? Are you nonthreatening and accepting, treating each learner as an individual? Do your teaching methods enhance learning by giving positive reinforcement to the learner? Are you aware of your nonverbal communication?

The following is a list of some principles of adult learning that, if taken into consideration by instructors, will greatly enhance the effectiveness of the presentations:

1. Instructional activities should be task-oriented whenever possible and include active participation by the learners. Adults should experience success in completing the activity and should be able to demonstrate the skill in new situations.

2. Adults need to see the achievement of what they have learned and the instructor needs to respond to achievement with positive acknowledgment and praise.

3. Teaching tools should be used that aid learners in discovering for themselves the gaps between where they are and where they want to be. Such tools include a self-directed learning plan, appraisal systems, and exposure to role models.

4. Because adults are usually ready to learn only things they need to know in order to cope effectively with real life situations, actual or simulated cases should be the focus of most teaching.

5. Learning should be problem-centered because that is how adults learn best.

6. Because of the learners' diverse backgrounds, adult learning requires an emphasis on individuation of teaching and learning strategies. Therefore, there should be an empha-

sis on experiential techniques—techniques that tap into the experiences of the learners, such as simulation exercises, problem-solving activities, case methods, and discussion.

7. The climate established in a classroom is based on verbal and nonverbal communication. What the teacher says can set a tone or pattern of interaction that can encourage or discourage learner participation. Dominant teacher talk, lack of praise, ignoring learners' ideas, criticizing, and not asking questions will inhibit learner involvement. Verbal statements that bring trainees into the discussion and involve them in interaction encourage adult learners to participate by making them feel an important part of the learning situation.

8. Nonverbal behavior by the teacher can also encourage or inhibit involvement by the adult trainee. Teacher-initiated moves, such as responding to a raised hand or a puzzled look, will build an effective learning climate. Expressions that support students, manifest approval, exhibit encouragement, and connote enjoyment or praise will aid more in climate building than expression of dissatisfaction, discouragement, or punishment.

9. Verbal expression and nonverbal movements send messages to trainees. It is important that these messages convey support, acceptance, responsiveness, and positive regard. The trainee does best when he or she feels secure.

TEACHING METHODS

To maintain interest by both the instructor and trainee in the educational process, different methods of teaching need to be used. Methods, such as lecture, audiovisuals, and group discussion, are the way the educational information is presented.

Lecture

Lecture is probably the teaching method most often used in the classroom, and usually the basic flow of information is from the instructor to the students. During a lecture more material can be covered in a short period of time. It is an effective way to provide an overview of material or present general information or facts. Student participation is limited with a lecture, so be alert to their receptivity and interject questions periodically.

Pointers:

- Rehearse the lecture.
- Change your voice volume and pace.
- Speak slowly and clearly.
- Take a deep breath before starting.
- Maintain eye contact.

Audiovisuals

Audiovisuals are an excellent way to supplement and enhance a presentation. Handouts, videotapes, slides, and overhead transparencies are examples of audiovisuals.
Pointers:

- Introduce the audiovisual. Do not assume it is self-explanatory.
- If showing a videotape, tell the trainees what you want them to be watching for.
- If using a videotape or overhead projector, check the screen from the trainees' seating area to make sure everyone has an unobstructed view.

(See Guidelines for Designing and Using Overhead Transparencies in this guide for more pointers on the use of overhead transparencies.)

Group Discussion

Group discussion is a free exchange of ideas among trainees. It is learner-centered and gives trainees the opportunity to convince themselves and solve problems.
Pointers:

- Initiate group discussion in groups with 12–15 people. If the group is too large, divide it into small groups.
- Open the discussion with a question or problem that will focus on the activity.
- End the discussion period with closure, such as a summary of what was discussed or a report from the group.

(See Questioning Techniques for more information on the use of questions.)

Case Studies

Case studies are a variation of group discussions. A case or situation is presented to the class either verbally, in writing, in pictures, or on videotape. The class, or small groups, are asked one or more questions about the case. This method is an excellent way to problem solve and it encourages everyone to participate.

Pointers:

- If a written case is presented, it should be short (about two paragraphs).
- Have the question(s) prepared in advance (e.g., "What would you do in this situation?" or "What should have been done in this situation?").

(See Questioning Techniques in this guide for more information on the use of questions.)

Role Play

Role play is the acting out of a situation or incident by the trainees. It is an effective way to teach insight into the feelings and roles of other people and the forces at play in certain situations.

Pointers:

- Give players time to prepare for their roles.
- Assign roles to all trainees even if they are not acting out the situation (e.g., ask certain trainees to monitor the reactions and behavior of each of the players or to develop post–role playing questions for the group based on the activity).
- Do not force someone to play a role; it can be a very threatening experience for some individuals.
- Watch the players for signs of discomfort.
- Allow time for "debriefing" (i.e., time for the players to share what they felt and time for them to "get out of" the role).

Questioning Techniques

The use of questions during a session can encourage exchanging and sharing adult views. Through the exchange of differing views, tolerance, understanding, and appreciation can be developed. Questioning enables the teacher to assess what adults already know as well as what they need to learn, and provides a way to explore and arouse adult interest and curiosity. From questions and answers, the teacher can detect the degree of interest in the topic being studied. Questioning can be used to encourage adult interest by posing viewpoints not yet explored.

Pointers:

- Make sure questions are clear and understandable.
- Make eye contact when asking a particular person a question.

Please remember to complete the Class Evaluation sheet shown below for each session.

Class Evaluation

Date_____

Topic_____

Instructor_____

Instructions: Please fill out this form after each session. Your evaluations of the instructor and content of presentation will help us improve our teaching techniques for future classes. Place a check in the appropriate box next to each numbered statement.

Instructor Evaluation

	Very effective	Effective	Adequate	Less than adequate	Poor
1. Clearly stated focus and purpose of presentation					
2. Well-organized presentation, emphasizing main points					
3. Spoke in an interesting and enjoyable style (e.g., explained technical terminology, used humor)					

Content of Presentation

	Very effective	Effective	Adequate	Less than adequate	Poor
1. Material presented was current					
2. Audiovisuals were appropriate					
3. Useful information that can be applied to my work					

Comments/Suggestions for Improvement

_____
_____
_____
_____
_____
_____

Class evaluation sheet to be completed after each session.

GUIDELINES FOR DESIGNING
AND USING OVERHEAD TRANSPARENCIES

A few tables and figures from the units have been adapted for use as transparencies, and they appear in Appendix B. Instructions for making transparencies appear in the introduction to Appendix B. To create transparencies with the information provided in Appendix B, follow the suggestions below.

- Plan on using only one transparency for every 5 minutes of delivery.
- Limit each overhead to *one main* idea.
- Use a minimum of words (i.e., seven words per line and seven lines per page).
- Use lower-case letters; they are easier to read than upper-case letters.
- Use larger type size for headlines than for the rest of the material. Use at least 24-point letters for headlines and 18-point for text.
- Use underlining, shading, or boxes to highlight key points.
- Use consistency in typeface and layout throughout the presentation.
- Center your overheads, leaving more white space on the top and bottom than on the sides.
- Place more space around a group of text or figures than between the items in the group.
- Enlarge information so it is readable on an overhead before copying onto the transparency.
- Use colored transparencies—yellow is the preferred color.
- Never put up a transparency you feel you should apologize for. Redesign it before the presentation.
- Mount the transparencies within cardboard frames.
- Use frame borders for notes.
- Cover the transparency with white paper and slowly slide the paper down to reveal the information on the transparency point by point.
- Use a pointer to indicate specific ideas as you are speaking.
- Read from and point to the transparency, not to the screen.

- Simplify complex drawings. Consider drawing them yourself while giving the presentation so that you draw at the same speed as the learning is taking place.

- Turn off the projector when the transparency is not needed.

Unit I

Overview of Dementia

Learning Objectives

1. To differentiate the terms delirium and dementia
2. To state the major causes of delirium and dementia
3. To describe differences between the changes associated with normal aging and with Alzheimer's disease
4. To explain the behavior and emotional changes that occur in the person with Alzheimer's disease

When talking about people in a state of confusion, it is sometimes implied that delirium and dementia mean the same thing. However, the two are very different in meaning especially when referring to people with Alzheimer's disease.

WHAT IS DELIRIUM?

Delirium refers to a group of symptoms that cause temporary impairment of mental function. It is not a normal part of aging. Symptoms include memory loss, emotional instability, loss of sense of time and place, possible hallucinations and/or delusions, and possible decreases in alertness and level of consciousness. Delirium may also be referred to as confusion. The onset of delirium is usually abrupt (within hours or a day) and always has a physical cause: infection, dehydration, poor nutrition, or reaction to medications. Confusion is caused by diseases and physical problems as well as environmental, psychological, and social conditions.

Delirium is likely to occur more in frail older people who have diminished ability to adapt to physical and/or environmental changes. It can occur alone or with dementia. If dementia is present, the person's ability to adapt to changes is decreased and the likelihood of delirium occurring with ill-ness rises.

Sundowning is a type of delirium. This is the term that is sometimes applied to confused behavior that occurs late in the afternoon or early evening. It is not clear why some people exhibit this behavior and some do not. Changes within and around the person cause the confused behavior to become worse. Such changes include the sun setting, rooms becoming dimly lit and making it difficult to discern objects clearly, activity level in the person's surroundings changes, normal alterations in the body rhythms that often raise body temperature and lower blood pressure, changes in blood sugar levels, and the cumulative effect of medications. If left untreated, the underlying cause may lead to permanent brain damage and cause dementia or increase existing dementia.

WHAT IS DEMENTIA?

Dementia refers to a loss of intellectual function (e.g., thinking, remembering, reasoning) of sufficient severity to interfere with an individual's daily functioning. Dementia is not a disease in itself but a group of symptoms that may accompany certain diseases or conditions. Symptoms may include changes in personality, mood, and behavior. Depression and dementia are most often confused. Table 1.1 delineates the differences between the two. Table 1.2 then compares the various features (e.g., onset, duration) of confusion/delirium, dementia, and depression.

True dementias are caused by diseases for which there are currently no cures, and are progressive and irreversible. The following are some diseases that are known to cause dementia.

Alzheimer's Disease

Alzheimer's disease is sometimes erroneously called senile dementia of the Alzheimer's type (SDAT), organic brain syndrome, or senile psychosis. It is a condition in which brain cells are damaged from the accumulation of neurofibrillary tangles and neuritic plaques or the loss of neurotransmitters. Alzheimer's disease is the most common of the dementing diseases, affecting as many as 4 million Americans thus far. The rate of progression varies from case to case. To date, there is no method of prevention and no cure. A new drug, tacrine, which was approved by the Food and Drug Administration in 1993, is

Table 1.1. Differences between depression and dementia

Depression	Dementia
Variable age	Elderly (usually)
Rapid onset	Gradual onset
Family aware	Family unaware (but sometimes suspicious)
Often cooperative	Often uncooperative
Sometimes past psychiatric history	Often no psychiatric history
Specific onset date	No specific date
Precipitating factors often present	No clear precipitant
CT scan/EEG usually normal	CT scan/EEG often abnormal
Emotional and cognitive symptoms	Often only cognitive symptoms
Specific Symptoms	
Rarely disoriented	Often disoriented
May appear confused	Often confused
Intellect preserved	Intellect lost
Affect depressed	Affect shallow
Possible diurnal variation	Sundowning (worse in afternoons)
Apathetic—doesn't try; "Don't know, don't care"	Tries to perform
Details symptoms	Vague complaints
Emphasizes disability	Minimizes, confabulates
Focuses on failures	Focuses on accomplishments
Concentration is variable	Concentration is variable
Decreased decision-making effort	Decreased decision-making ability
Decreased recent and remote memory	Decreased recent and variable remote memory
Inconsistent poor performance	Fairly consistent poor performance
Rarely perseverates	More often perseverates
Occasionally suicidal	Rarely suicidal
Self-esteem often low	Self-esteem often okay
Appetite often changed	Appetite usually okay
Energy often reduced	Energy often okay
Sleep often disturbed	Sleep often okay
Feels like "I never was"	Feels like "I used to be"

proving helpful in slowing the progression of symptoms in some people.

Creutzfeldt-Jakob Disease (CJD)

Creutzfeldt-Jakob disease is a rare fatal brain disease caused by a transmissible infectious agent, probably a slow virus, (i.e., a virus that does not manifest itself for years after it is acquired). Failing memory, changes in behavior, and lack of co-ordination are some of the symptoms observed in the early stages of the disease. Creutzfeldt-Jakob disease progresses rapidly, causing mental deterioration, involuntary muscle

Table 1.2.   Clinical features of confusion/delirium, dementia, and depression

Feature	Confusion/delirium	Dementia	Depression
Onset	Acute/subacute, depends on cause	Chronic, generally subtle, depends on cause	Coincides with life changes, often abrupt
Course	Short, diurnal fluctuations in symptoms, worse at night, dark, and on awakening	Long, no diurnal effects, symptoms progressive yet relatively stable over time	Diurnal effects, typically worse in the morning; situational fluctuations
Duration	Hours to less than 1 month	Months to years	At least 2 weeks, can be several months or years
Alertness	Fluctuates	Generally normal	Normal
Orientation	Fluctuates in severity, generally impaired	May be impaired	Selective disorientation
Memory	Recent and immediate impaired	Recent and remote impaired	Selective or patchy impairment
Thinking	Disorganized, distorted, fragmented, slow, or accelerated	Difficulty with abstraction	Intact
Perception	Distorted, illusions, delusions	Misperceptions often absent	Variable hallucinations
Psychomotor behavior	Variable, hypokinetic, hyperkinetic, or mixed	Variable	Normal or minimally hypokinetic
Sleep-wake cycle	Disturbed, cycle reversed	Fragmented	Disturbed
EEG	Related to state of arousal	Normal or slow	Normal
Mini-Mental Status Exam	Mean score, 12	Mean score, 7	Mean score, 19
Associated features	Variable affective changes, symptoms of autonomic hyperarousal	Affect tends to be superficial, inappropriate, and labile	Affect depressed, dysphoric mood exaggerated and detailed complaints

jerks, and generalized weakness. The person with the disease may become blind and eventually lapse into a coma. Death usually occurs within 1 year after diagnosis. Examination of brain tissue reveals distinct cellular changes unlike those seen in Alzheimer's disease. No treatment is currently available to stop the progression of the disease.

Huntington's Disease (HD)

Huntington's disease is a hereditary disorder that usually begins in mid-life and is characterized by irregular involuntary movements of the limbs or facial muscles and a decline in intellectual processes. Psychiatric problems are common, with depression and memory disturbances occurring in early stages. The pattern of memory impairment differs from that seen in Alzheimer's disease. As Huntington's disease progresses, movements become severe and uncontrollable; mental capacity may deteriorate to dementia.

A family history of the disease and the recognition of typical movement disorders and brain scanning provide evidence for a diagnosis of Huntington's disease. A genetic marker linked to the Huntington gene has been identified on chromosome 4. Researchers have been working to locate the gene itself. The movement disorders and psychiatric symptoms seen in Huntington's disease can be somewhat controlled or lessened by prescribed medications; however, no treatment is available to stop the progression of the disease.

Multiple Infarct Dementia (MID)

Multiple infarct dementia is caused by blood vessel disease that results in mini strokes, or *little strokes,* causing progressive damage to the brain cells. The onset of MID may be relatively sudden. These strokes may damage areas of the brain responsible for a specific function, such as calculations, and there may be more generalized symptoms, such as disorientation, confusion, and behavior changes. A person may develop localized neurological deficits and experience trouble swallowing, problems with speech, or paralysis in an extremity. Multiple infarct dementia may appear similar to Alzheimer's disease and the two co-exist in 15%–20% of people with dementia.

Brain scanning techniques are used to identify strokes. Computerized tomography (CT scan) and magnetic resonance imaging (MRI) are two scanning techniques. If these *little strokes* have occurred, the radiologist can see these areas on the brain scan. Multiple infarct dementia progresses in downhill steps with periods of stability and possibly some slight improvement between strokes.

Histories of high blood pressure, vascular disease, diabetes, or previous strokes have been identified as risk factors of multiple infarct dementia. It is not reversible nor curable; however, recognition of an underlying condition, such as hypertension, often leads to specific treatment that may halt the progression of the disorder. Sometimes an aspirin taken daily is prescribed as a prevention.

Multiple Sclerosis

Multiple sclerosis is a disease of unknown cause that usually begins before the age of 40. The causative agent, possibly a virus, causes damage to the protective myelin covering on nerve cells. This results in physical damage (e.g., imbalance, gait disturbance, muscle weakness) and eventual mental deterioration. The course of the disease may be manifested in rapid deterioration of the person, or there may be periods of remission and exacerbation. Eventually there may be memory loss and disorientation.

Normal Pressure Hydrocephalus (NPH)

Normal pressure hydrocephalus is an uncommon disease in older people that is characterized by difficulty in walking, dementia, and urinary incontinence. An obstruction in the normal flow of the spinal fluid causes the fluid to build up, thus creating pressure on the brain structure that results in degenerative changes (e.g., memory loss, confusion, unsteady balance). Presently the most useful diagnostic tool is the MRI scan. Possible contributing factors may be a history of meningitis, encephalitis, or head trauma. In addition to treatment of the underlying cause, the condition may be corrected by a neurosurgical procedure (shunt) to divert fluid outside the brain.

Parkinson's Disease

Parkinson's disease is a condition in which an important neurotransmitter of the brain called dopamine, which is involved in the control of muscle activity by the nervous system, is inadequately produced. Characteristics of Parkinson's disease include tremor, stiffness, slowness, and slow speech. Difficulty in swallowing and a tendency to choke also occur. Late in the course of the disease, some people develop dementia. Some people with Parkinson's disease develop Alzheimer's disease and some people with Alzheimer's disease develop symptoms of Parkinson's disease. Medications for Parkinson's disease can improve the motor skill symptoms, but they do not improve the mental changes that occur. Medications such as levodopa, which converts itself into dopamine once inside the brain, and deprenyl, which prevents degeneration of dopamine-containing neurons, are the most frequently used. Parkinson's disease frequently serves as a model for drug research on Alzheimer's disease.

Pick's Disease

Pick's disease is a rare brain disease that closely resembles Alzheimer's disease and is usually difficult to diagnose clinically. Disturbances in personality, behavior, and orientation may precede and initially be more severe than memory defects. As in Alzheimer's disease, a definitive diagnosis is usually obtained at autopsy.

Other Conditions

There are a number of conditions that cause dementia-like symptoms: depression, drug reactions, thyroid disorders, nutritional deficiencies, brain tumors, head injuries, alcoholism, infections (e.g., meningitis, syphilis, acquired immunodeficiency syndrome). Symptoms caused by these conditions are called *pseudodementia* or false dementia. It is important that these conditions be ruled out during medical diagnostics as the dementia from these conditions may be slowed or stopped with treatment. A definition of terms related to dementia is shown in Table 1.3.

WHAT HAPPENS IN DEMENTIA?

Whatever the underlying disease, dementia is caused by damage to nerve cells in the brain, which causes behavior changes. As the disease progresses, the damage gets progressively worse and more function is lost.

Nerve cells in the brain have three basic functions: *storing information, using or processing information,* and *transmitting information.* When cells are damaged, information once stored may become unavailable or simply lost to the person (e.g., he or she may get lost in a familiar neighborhood or be unable to name a familiar object).

When cells can no longer use or process information, the individual has difficulty making judgments or understanding task sequence or the results of actions (e.g., he or she may dress with underwear on the outside of pants, become flustered trying to decide which eating utensil to use, or overreact to a situation and strike out).

When cells stop transmitting information, the person starts losing voluntary control over his or her body (e.g., inability to walk, sit up straight, and swallow).

Table 1.3.   Mental status changes: A definition of terms

Affect   A subjectively experienced feeling, state, or emotion that is expressed by observable behavior.

Agnosia   Inability to recognize or understand either sounds or speech.

Aphasia   Problems understanding words or remembering particular words; may be expressive, receptive, or both.

Apraxia   Difficulty knowing how to manipulate or use common objects.

Catastrophic reaction   An extreme reaction to a situation that occurs when people with dementia become very upset or overwhelmed.

Concentration   The effortful, deliberate, and heightened state of attention in which irrelevant stimuli are deliberately excluded from conscious awareness.

Confusion   A mental state in which reactions to environmental stimuli are inappropriate; person is bewildered or perplexed or unable to orientate him- or herself. Same as delirium if onset is sudden.

Constructional praxis   The capacity to draw or construct 2- or 3-dimensional figures or shapes.

Delirium   A *sudden onset* mental status change that has an organic cause.

Delusion   A false belief or wrong judgment held with conviction despite incontrovertible evidence to the contrary.

Dementia   A debilitating condition of the brain caused by various diseases and characterized by loss of memory, function, and personality.

Depression   An ongoing sadness that may accompany dementia, especially in early stages of dementia; can be caused by other physical disease entities (e.g., hypothyroidism).

Hallucination   The apparent, often strong subjective perception of an object or event when no such situation is present.

Insight   The ability of a person to observe him- or herself and a situation and to interpret this observation in a way that is consistent with the perceptions of others.

Judgment   The ability to recognize social situations and the socially appropriate or safe response in such situations and to apply the correct response when faced with the real situation.

Mood   A pervasive and sustained emotion that may markedly color a person's perception of the world (e.g., depression, anxiety, elation).

Orientation   Awareness of where one is in relation to time, place, person, and situation.

Paranoia   A false belief that one is going to be harmed in some way by someone or something.

Paraphasia   A form of aphasia in which the person has lost the power to speak correctly (e.g., substituting one word for another and jumbling words and sentences in such a way as to make speech unintelligible).

Perception   The intellectual function that integrates sensory impressions into meaningful data and to memory. Perceptual functions include such activities as awareness, recognition, discrimination, patterning, and orientation.

Sundowning   Confusion that often occurs in the late afternoon or night.

Visual agnosia   The inability to understand what one is seeing (e.g., seeing a table but not being able to recognize it as a table).

The person with Alzheimer's disease is not responsible for his or her behavior! Damage to the brain cells has made information storage, processing, and transmission impossible and the damage will only get worse as the disease progresses.

WHAT IS ALZHEIMER'S DISEASE?

Alzheimer's disease or the grouping of characteristics that we attribute to Alzheimer's disease is distinguished from other forms of dementia by characteristic changes in the brain that are visible only upon microscopic examination. At autopsy, brains of people with Alzheimer's disease show the presence of tangles of fibers (i.e., neurofibrillary tangles) and clusters of degenerative nerve endings (i.e., neuritic plaques) in areas that are important for memory and intellectual functions. Recently, advances in anatomic and physiologic imaging techniques (computer axial tomography [CAT] and magnetic resonance imaging [MRI]) of living brains have begun to document some changes that commonly occur in the brains of people with Alzheimer's disease (e.g., enlargement of the temporal horn and Sylvian fissure in the brain, as well as larger cerebrospinal fluid volumes and smaller overall brain volumes). Figure 1.1 shows the physical differences between the brain of a person with Alzheimer's disease and the brain of a person without Alzheimer's disease. Figure 1.2 shows neurofibrillary changes in the brain of a person with Alzheimer's disease can also be compared.

Another occurrence of Alzheimer's disease is the reduced production of certain brain chemicals, especially acetylcholine and somatostatin. These chemicals are necessary for normal communication among nerve cells.

Alzheimer's disease is more likely to occur as a person gets older and is found more frequently in women than in men. Approximately 10% of people over age 65 have Alzheimer's disease. This percentage rises to 47% in those over age 85. It can occur in middle age as well, although onset before the age of 60 is rare. The youngest documented case is that of a 28-year-old individual.

WHAT CAUSES ALZHEIMER'S DISEASE?

There are three major theories for the cause(s) of Alzheimer's disease. The first one and the one that pharmaceutical companies are utilizing for treatment research is the *neurotransmitter theory*. Neurotransmitters such as dopamine, acetylcholine, and serotonin are substances in the brain that are necessary for messages to be carried from one nerve to another. They are important in learning and memory. This theory suggests that

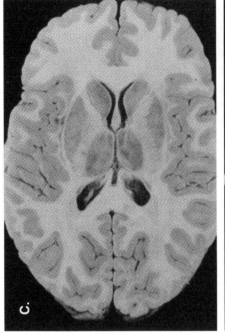

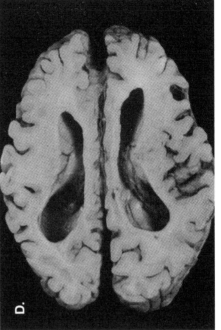

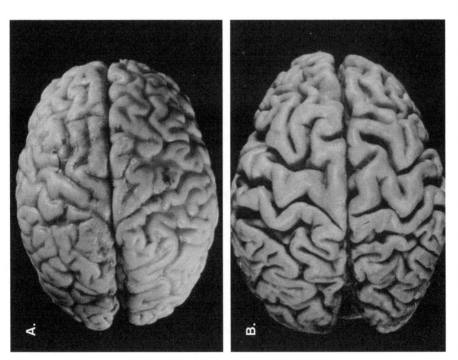

Figure 1.1. (A) Human brain of a person without Alzheimer's disease; (B) Human brain of a person with Alzheimer's disease (Note atrophic surface area lost by decrease in gyri and deeper, wider sulci;); (C) Section of a human brain of a person without Alzheimer's disease; (D) Section of a human brain of a person with Alzheimer's disease (Note the enlarged ventricles.). (From Gwyther, L.P. [1985]. *Care of Alzheimer's patients: A manual for nursing home staff*. Washington, DC: American Health Care Association and the Alzheimer's Association; reprinted by permission.)

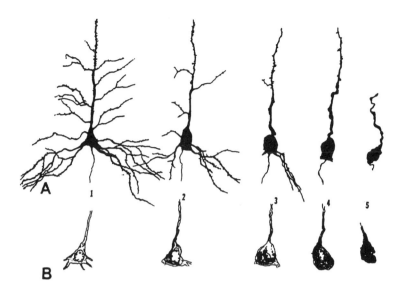

Figure 1.2.   (A) Progressive changes in neurons with aging in a person without Alzheimer's disease, (B) Appearance of neurons showing neurofibrillary changes in a person with Alzheimer's disease. (From Scheibel, M.E., Nandy, K., & Sherwin, I. [1977]. *The aging brain and senile dementia.* New York: Plenum; reprinted by permission.)

the production of neurotransmitters is reduced in people with Alzheimer's disease.

The second theory is based on *genetics*. It is widely known that people born with Down syndrome will very likely experience a dementia similar to Alzheimer's disease by the age of 40 or 45. Down syndrome is caused by a defect on chromosome 21. Scientists have also found a similar defect on chromosome 4. Familial Alzheimer's disease of early onset (before the age of 60 years) is associated with abnormal changes in the protein amyloid beta. This protein may be deposited in the brain of people with Alzheimer's disease, and is found on chromosomes 21 and 14. Late-onset familial Alzheimer's disease and sporadically occurring Alzheimer's disease have been linked to another protein, apoliprotein-E4. This is a normal, cholesterol-carrying protein that, if genetically influenced, can interact in an abnormal way with amyloid beta protein and play a role in the development of Alzheimer's disease. Apoliprotein-E4 is associated with chromosome 19.

Exposure to aluminum salts is the basis for the *toxin theory*. These salts are present in drinking water, foods, cooking utensils, and buffered antacids. A few investigators have reported higher concentrations of aluminum in the brains of people with Alzheimer's disease than in those of healthy older people. This theory is yet to be validated.

WHAT ARE THE SYMPTOMS OF ALZHEIMER'S DISEASE?

Alzheimer's disease has a gradual onset. Symptoms include difficulty with memory and loss of intellectual abilities severe enough to interfere with daily routines or social activities. People with Alzheimer's disease may also experience confusion, language problems (e.g., trouble finding words), poor or decreased judgment, and changes in personality and behavior. How quickly these changes occur varies from person to person. Alzheimer's disease eventually leaves people unable to care for themselves. From the time symptoms first appear, Alzheimer's disease lasts about 8 years; however, it has been known to last as long as 25 years. The progression of Alzheimer's disease can be described in three stages.

First Stage

The first stage of Alzheimer's disease lasts between 2 and 4 years and includes the period leading up to and including diagnosis. One of the first symptoms is recent memory loss. Symptoms are often overlooked or dismissed as a result of stress or illness. The individual may be the first to notice a problem while family and friends begin noticing subtle changes.

The signs and symptoms of the first stage may include the following:

- Progressive forgetfulness (e.g., has difficulty with routine chores, loses items and forgets they are lost)
- Confusion about directions, decisions, and money management (e.g., gets lost in his or her own neighborhood, forgets to pay bills)
- Loss of spontaneity and initiative (e.g., loses spark or zest for life, is less outgoing, has difficulty starting anything)
- Repetition of actions and statements (e.g., repeats things; engages in continuous activities such as lip smacking, chewing, tapping, or saying a word or phrase over and over)
- Change in mood or personality (e.g., denies forgetfulness, accuses others of hiding things)
- Disorientation of time and place (e.g., shows up for appointments at wrong time or place, constantly checks the calendar)

Second Stage

The second stage of Alzheimer's disease is the longest stage, lasting from 2 to 12 years after diagnosis. Symptoms are evident, and it is obvious that the person has Alzheimer's disease. The second stage can be divided into early and late stages based on degree of dependency.

The signs and symptoms of the second stage may include the following:

- Difficulty recognizing close friends and family and knowing socially acceptable behavior
- Inability to retain new experiences
- Tendency to wander
- Restlessness, especially in late afternoon and evening
- Occasional muscle twitching or jerking
- Difficulty organizing thoughts (e.g., vocabulary is markedly diminished, can speak but selection of words may not make sense, cannot comprehend writing)
- Irritability, tendency to be fidgety or teary, insensitivity (Catastrophic reactions and sleep disturbances may begin at this stage.)
- Sloppiness and confusion about dressing—needs assistance with all daily care activities
- Incontinence because of inability to find the toilet or communicate need
- Hallucinations (i.e., seeing or hearing things that are not there)
- Increased need for oral stimulation (e.g., will eat or chew on anything available; forgets when last meal was eaten, then loses interest)

Third Stage

The third stage of Alzheimer's disease lasts 1–3 years and ends in death. The most recognizable symptom is that the person is unable to recognize family members or him- or herself in the mirror.

The signs and symptoms of the third stage may include the following:

- Weight loss even with proper diet and eventual emaciation
- Inability to perform any daily care activities, total dependence, and incontinence

- Inability to communicate and obliviousness to environment
- Extreme irritability
- Increased need for oral stimulation
- Inability to walk or sit up
- Increased need for sleep, which leads to coma

People with Alzheimer's disease usually die from pneumonia or other infections. Accidents, malnutrition, and dehydration often contribute to death.

HOW IS ALZHEIMER'S DISEASE DIAGNOSED?

About 10%–20% of all dementias are the result of treatable problems, including depression, and are not true dementias at all. Of the remaining dementias that are treatable, 60% result from Alzheimer's disease, 20% from multiple infarct dementia, and about 20% from both.

Diagnosis begins with eliminating treatable causes of dementia. This is a difficult and lengthy process that consists largely of determining what the patient does not have rather than what he or she does have.

The examination to determine Alzheimer's disease should include a detailed medical history, mental status test, neuropsychological testing, blood work, urinalysis, chest x-ray, electroencephalogram (EEG), computerized tomography (CT scan), and electrocardiogram (ECG). This kind of an evaluation will determine whether the dementia is the result of a treatable illness such as hypothyroidism, electrolyte imbalance, infection, anemia, medication toxicity, brain tumor, or any other condition.

When this detailed examination is done, the accuracy of diagnosis is about 90%. However, the only way to confirm a diagnosis of Alzheimer's disease is to examine brain tissue under a microscope after the person has died.

WHAT MEDICAL TREATMENT CAN BE GIVEN?

Medical treatment of delirium involves the elimination or treatment of the underlying cause such as changing medications, rehydrating and feeding the individual, treating an infection, or assisting with adjustment to a new environment. Because depression often mimics delirium and/or dementia and is usually treatable, it is essential that depression be identified, if present, and treated appropriately.

Medical treatment of dementia is most often aimed at symptom control because the underlying causes are not curable. Medications to improve memory or cognitive abilities have had limited success with changes primarily seen only on cognitive tests and very little in the person's behavior.

Currently, there is only one medication, tacrine (Cognex), that shows real promise for slowing the progress of Alzheimer's disease. During its research stage it was referred to as tetrahydroacridine (THA). Tacrine slows down the deterioration in memory and improves an individual's ability to perform activities of daily living (ADLs). It must be offered to people with Alzheimer's disease in the early stages of the disease before functions are lost. If the person is already unable to perform activities of daily living or remember his or her name, the administration of tacrine will not bring back these functions. Eventually, the disease will progress beyond tacrine's ability to help, but function can be maintained for months or years. The disadvantages of tacrine are its side effects and high cost. One of the side effects is liver damage. Liver functions can be monitored and tacrine can be discontinued if necessary. Another side effect is gastrointestinal upset. Often individuals experiencing this side effect will discontinue taking tacrine with or without the physician's involvement. The cost of tacrine per month is much less than the cost of a month's stay in a nursing home.

Other medications are used to help manage some of the most troubling symptoms of Alzheimer's disease. Depression, behavior disturbance, and sleeplessness usually can be helped. Physical exercise, social activity, and proper nutrition and health maintenance are important for helping a person with Alzheimer's disease maintain a fulfilling and comfortable life.

UNIT 1: QUIZ

Please take a few minutes to complete the quiz for this unit. Answer each question as best you can. Keep in mind this is a learning tool to help you summarize and remember what has been discussed in this unit. For true-false questions, check the correct answer. For multiple choice questions, circle the correct answer(s).

Note: There may be more than one correct answer for some questions.

1. Alzheimer's disease is:

   a. A brain disorder that cannot be controlled.

   b. A normal part of aging.

   c. Easily diagnosable.

   d. None of the above.

2. A person with normal forgetfulness:

   a. Recalls that it is the Fourth of July when he or she sees fireworks.

   b. Remembers to keep a doctor's appointment because there is a note on the calendar.

   c. Forgets to find his or her glasses before reading the paper and cannot figure out why he or she cannot see the words.

   d. Cannot remember what he or she was looking for in the refrigerator.

3. People with Alzheimer's disease usually die from the effects of another condition or infection such as pneumonia.

   ____ True   ____ False

4. All people with Alzheimer's disease lose their abilities in the same manner.

    ____ True   ____ False

5. Which of the following statements describe people in the first stage of Alzheimer's disease?

    a. The person has some difficulty with recent memory such as events and names.

    b. The person may have difficulty concentrating and is absent-minded.

    c. Subtle personality changes may occur and the person may become depressed.

    d. The person is able to verbalize ideas and understand the ideas of others.

6. The following are characteristic forms of behavior for people in the second stage of dementia *except:*

    a. Loses all recent and some remote past memories including socially acceptable behavior.

    b. Easily makes decisions.

    c. Loses coordination and balance.

    d. Has increased agitation with pacing, wandering, and night wandering.

UNIT 1: INSTRUCTOR HELP

1. Preparation

    Have the room set up and materials ready before the participants are scheduled to arrive. This helps reduce anxiety.

2. Audiovisuals

    a. You may begin or end this session with the University of Washington videotape, "Overview Part I: Alzheimer's Disease and Related Disorders." This tape is 17 minutes long, so include this time in your lesson plan if you wish to use it.

    b. Four transparencies are provided for this session in Appendix B to assist in discussion. They include a figure of the brain, figure of neurons, definitions of terms, and three stages of Alzheimer's disease.

    c. Try to have a blackboard, whiteboard, newsprint pad on an easel, or something that you can utilize to write down ideas and questions that trainees may have.

    d. There are three tables for this session. They are for the trainees to use for reference after the course is completed.

3. Discussion/questions

    a. Open the session by asking the trainees what they think Alzheimer's disease is. Write down their responses. Come back to these responses at the end of the session and see if the responses have changed.

    b. After the trainees have answered the questions to the quiz, discuss the answers.

    c. Another way to begin the session is to utilize one of the handouts such as "Definition of Terms" and review the definitions of some of the more pertinent words. There is a transparency with portions of this table.

Unit 2

Communication

Learning Objectives

1. To differentiate between verbal and nonverbal communication and to discuss the importance of both

2. To demonstrate basic strategies for effective communication, such as maintaining eye contact, touching, stating ideas in positive terms, and using appropriate tone and inflection

3. To describe strategies for dealing with specific communication problems, such as word finding, repetitive questions, and making up information (i.e., when a person cannot remember what he or she is trying to say)

4. To describe the general deterioration of communication abilities from the early stages of Alzheimer's disease through the late stages

There are three basic steps of communication:

1. Production of an idea, which may or may not require using words

2. The expression of that idea through words and emotions

3. Reception and comprehension of that idea by another person

Ideas are expressed on two levels of communication. The first level is verbal or cognitive. This level is largely intentional communication; that is, individuals are aware of the words they use to express the idea. The nonverbal or emotional level is largely unintentional communication. Individuals are usually unaware of their body language, voice tone, and voice quality, which express the emotional component of their ideas. Table 2.1 shows the differences between verbal and nonverbal communication.

Table 2.1.   Communicating with people with Alzheimer's disease

Verbal Communication

1. Dialogue
    *   Use simple words.
    *   Use simple sentences.
    *   Give one command at a time.
    *   Do not use pronouns (e.g., he, she, it, they); use the name of the person or article.
    *   Repeat a question or command exactly as stated the first time.
    *   Always get a person's attention by calling his or her name.

2. Style
    *   Do not whisper.
    *   Use face-to-face communication, making sure the person can see your facial expressions and body language. Never use an intercom to call people with dementia.
    *   Do not speak louder than usual unless the person has a hearing impairment.
    *   Speak slowly.
    *   Speak in a quiet and calm voice.
    *   Minimize environmental stimuli.

Nonverbal Communication

*   Maintain eye contact. Touch the person gently.
*   Exaggerate facial expressions, gestures, and body movements.
*   Use a calm, gentle, and consistent approach no matter what the personal feelings.

Ideas and the words that express ideas can be very different. It is important to remember that the idea can exist separately from the word. Words are learned through a variety of associations, and although the word may not be remembered, the idea may be retained.

CHANGES IN COMMUNICATION ABILITIES IN PEOPLE WITH ALZHEIMER'S DISEASE

People with dementia gradually lose the ability to communicate meaningfully because they lose the ability to retrieve and use words to organize, express, and understand written or spoken ideas. They may retain most of their physical abilities involved in speech and reading and the nonverbal ability to communicate, produce, and understand emotions through body language.

When dementia is *mild,* communication problems are often overlooked because listeners assume mistakes are the result of fatigue, nervousness, or distraction, all of which can contribute to communication errors in people without dementia. Communication problems most commonly associated with mild dementia are the following:

• Shrinking vocabulary

• Frequent irrelevant comments

• Continuous repetitive words and movements (e.g., licking, lip smacking)

• Difficulty verbalizing ideas (e.g., trouble interpreting what is said or read)

In the early stages of dementia, the person usually is able to retain the mechanical aspects of speaking and reading (e.g., can read from a newspaper easily and speak sentences that sound correct). There usually is an ability to express a complete range of emotions and comprehend nonverbal emotional cues. Most people are also able to recognize and self-correct mistakes in speech.

When dementia becomes *moderately severe,* communication problems are more obvious and are rarely dismissed as normal. Communication problems most commonly associated with moderately severe dementia are the following:

• Difficulty naming objects, people, and events

• Inability to comprehend what is read

• Progressively shrinking vocabulary

• Difficulty reasoning aloud

The person usually retains the mechanical aspects of speaking or reading (e.g., may be able to read from a newspaper or speak sentences that sound correct, but word selection may not make sense). There is some ability to recognize and self-correct mistakes in speech. Complete emotional expression and comprehension of nonverbal cues are also retained.

When dementia is *severe,* communication problems are very obvious and often quite significant. A person may appear mute and unable to respond to any verbal communication attempts. Communication problems most commonly associated with severe dementia are the following:

• Extreme difficulty or inability to name objects, persons, events

• Extreme difficulty understanding spoken or written words

• Extreme difficulty writing or verbalizing

- Extremely limited vocabulary
- Inability to self-correct errors in speaking
- Possible appearance of muteness

Even with severe dementia, a person may be able to repeat sounds or generate an occasional correct phrase, but the meaning is lost. He or she may be able to say hello clearly when someone shakes his or her hand but the meaning is lost. Most important to remember is the fact that even people with severe dementia retain the ability to comprehend nonverbal emotional cues as well as express emotions. At this stage of Alzheimer's disease, nonverbal communication is the most important. The speaker's body language and voice tone should match the words.

The article, "I've Lost a Kingdom: A Victim's Remarks on Alzheimer's Disease," is provided in the unit appendix. Marguerite R. Lerner's comments over a 2-year period painfully and clearly evidence the thoughts of a person with Alzheimer's disease.

COMMUNICATION TECHNIQUES

Communication with people with Alzheimer's disease is more effective when caregivers remember the progression of losses and utilize retained abilities. The following are suggested general guidelines for improving communication techniques with people with Alzheimer's disease:

1. Evaluate hearing and vision, if possible. Do this before assuming that communication problems are the direct result of dementia. This can be difficult if the person cannot understand what is happening. Sometimes a family member or caregiver who knows the person can provide some information regarding hearing and vision changes. If hearing or vision aids are available, be sure they are in working order and are used.

2. Improve your listening skills. If the person is verbalizing at all, he or she is trying to communicate. Take time to listen and show interest.

   - Be patient and give the person time to respond.
   - Do not interrupt the person or argue with him or her.
   - Be sure you understand what the person is saying.

- Remember that the person will forget what was just said and the message will need to be repeated.
- Watch the person's body language to determine readiness for communication. By identifying nonreceptive behavior, strong negative reactions (i.e., catastrophic reactions) may be avoided. Nonreceptive behavior includes backing away, turning the head or body away, shrinking away from touch, avoiding eye contact, pulling away, frowning, increased body tension, fidgeting, shaking, increased respiratory/heart rate, flushed or pale skin color, narrowed or closed eyes, and a higher pitched voice. When the person is nonreceptive, tell him or her that you understand he or she is not ready to talk now, and will return later. Be sure to return as this will demonstrate commitment to the person and help establish trust.

3. Improve the time and place of communication. When communicating with a person, make sure you are in a place that, at the time, has no other activities going on that may distract the person.

- Approach the person from the front, never from behind.
- Always identify yourself to the person.
- Be sure to have the person's undivided attention. Be certain he or she can see you. Use more than one of the five senses to get the person's attention. Call the person's name, touch him or her on the shoulder, or take his or her hand; or allow your body stance to imitate or mirror that of the person.
- Place your face in the person's direct line of vision whether he or she is standing, sitting in a wheelchair, or lying in bed.
- Be sure your face is fully illuminated; the light from the window or lamp should be behind the person, not behind you.
- Reduce all background noise and distractions. Move to a quieter area if necessary.
- Allow enough time for the communication to take place.

4. Improve your self-expression during communication.

- Match the emotional content of communication (i.e., nonverbal behavior) with the verbal content.

- Learn to analyze the emotional content of communication from the point of view of the person.

5. Think before speaking, plan how to communicate as well as what to say.

   - Anticipate problems that will occur and have alternate strategies ready.
   - Explain what will be done before doing it.
   - Assume the person always hears what is said (i.e., don't say anything in front of the person that you do not wish him or her to hear).

6. Facilitate communication.

   - Adjust your speed and complexity of words and sentences to the person's level of ability. Limit sentences and questions to one step or one idea at a time, if needed.
   - Help with word finding by offering two alternate choices; do not correct the person.
   - Avoid using abstract words, generalizations, and pronouns because these are too complex for the person to understand (e.g., Do not say "Here it is"; say "Here is your coat.").
   - Modify questions to avoid open-ended questions. Instead, use yes/no and either/or questions (e.g., Do not ask "What would you like to drink?"; ask "Would you like water or juice to drink?").
   - Be redundant. Repeat the sentence or question exactly at least once. If that fails, restate the question using other related words that the person may understand (e.g., Ask "Would you like water or orange juice?" pause, then repeat "Would you like water or orange juice?" pause, then ask "Are you thirsty?").
   - Use right-branching sentences rather than left-branching sentences. Left-branching sentences require the listener to remember the left half of the sentence (first half) in order to understand the right half (last part) of sentence. For example, "Would you like water or orange juice to drink?" is a left-branching sentence. The person hears the choices before the question and must remember them to be able to reply. "Would you like to drink water or orange juice?" is a right-branching sentence and does not require the same degree of mental processing to respond.

- Be direct and explicit about what you mean (e.g., If you are busy with another person, do not say "I'm working with Mary now" but say, "I cannot talk with you now. I will talk with you later.").

- Avoid abstract discussions.

- Avoid using analogies. The type of language processing required to understand analogies is extremely complex and is very difficult for people with dementia.

It is important to remember that even though the individual with Alzheimer's disease has difficulty communicating, he or she continues to experience feelings, such as joy, sadness, fear, and anger. Figure 2.1 gives helpful suggestions for communicating with people with Alzheimer's disease in ways that are considerate of their feelings. Figure 2.2 offers two role-playing situations that are good exercise in practicing communication techniques.

Alzheimer's disease affects a person's ability to think, communicate, and perform the basic activities of daily living. But like people of all ages, the Alzheimer patient experiences feelings of joy, sadness, fear, anger, and jealousy. As a caregiver, you need to recognize and respond to these feelings. A person with this disease needs to feel valued, worthwhile, and positive about life.

Like many people in their later years, the person with Alzheimer's disease must cope with and adjust to many changes—from body image and retirement, to shifts in lifestyle and preparation for disability and death. Many people also look back over their lives and try to make sense of what they've accomplished. Often, for example, they review past relationships and try to make amends.

The caregiver can learn to help the person with Alzheimer's disease deal with these issues by understanding the person's reactions to the effects of the disease. You can assist the family member in dealing with feelings by exercising patience, sensitivity, a sense of humor, and by using the following steps:

ACTION STEPS

Treat the "Patient" as a Person

- Appreciate and acknowledge the Alzheimer patient as a person. Through words and touch, try to do everything you can to relate to this individual as a valued human being with emotional and spiritual needs.

- Avoid talking about the person. People with Alzheimer's disease are often hurt when caregivers talk about them as if they're in another room. Typical are such comments as these:

  - "She's giving us a lot of trouble."

  - "Yesterday was a bad time for her."

  - "She kept me up all night again."

  Instead of talking about the person, assume that she understands everything you're saying.

- Call the person with Alzheimer's disease by his or her name. Avoid cruel and dehumanizing descriptions such as "the bedwetter," "gramps," or "granny." Also avoid isolating the individual from visitors.

Communicate Slowly and Calmly

- Speak slowly and in simple sentences. Slow down your rate of speech and lower the pitch of your voice.

- Give the person with Alzheimer's time to hear your words and prepare a response. Keep in mind that it can take up to a minute for the person with this disease to respond.

- Keep communication on an adult-to-adult level. Avoid baby talk or demeaning expressions. Smiles and handshakes go a long way to set the tone for adult interactions.

- Communicate one message at a time. The person with Alzheimer's disease can become confused by a long string of messages such as: "Good morning. Let's get dressed and come down and eat our breakfast." Instead, divide the message into sections such as:

  - "Good morning. You need to get up now."

  - "OK, you're up. Now let's get dressed."

  - "OK, why don't we go downstairs now?"

  - "It's time for breakfast."

- Keep in mind that the person with Alzheimer's disease probably can't tell time. Instead of saying, "John will be here at 2 o'clock," say, "John will be here after your bath."

(continued)

Figure 2.1.   Guidelines for handling feelings. (From Alzheimers's Disease and Related Disorders Association, Inc. [1990]. *Feelings*. Chicago: Author; reprinted by permission.)

Figure 2.1   *(continued)*

Be Positive and Reassuring

- Be positive, optimistic and reassuring to the person. Use such expressions as "Everything will be OK. Don't worry. We're doing great. We're going to get through this. I'm here to help you." Expressing your feelings will help you release tension and help comfort the person.

- Use comforting and non-controlling statements. Try to identify feelings rather than argue about facts. For example, instead of arguing with the person about going outside, you can agree by saying, "Yes, it would be fun to go outside." Or put limits on the request by saying, "I want to go outside, too. Let's do it after we eat. I'm hungry!" As an alternative, you can distract the person by saying, "Yes, it's nice to go outside. That's a nice sweater you're wearing."

- Give praise for the simplest achievements and successes by making such comments as, "That's great," "You're doing really well," or "Oh, you did such a good job with that."

Tell the Person What to Expect

- Prepare the person for what's about to happen. Instead of pulling the patient out of a chair or pushing the patient across the room, make such comments as, "We need to get up now." Then, gently assist the person to get out of the chair or move across the room.

- Provide suggestions and structure. For example, don't ask, "Do you want to take a bath?" Instead, say, "It's time to take your bath now."

Situation #1

Mrs. Jones is 70 years old. She has Alzheimer's disease and is very confused. She is living in your care facility.

Player #1: Mrs. Jones

It is 3 A.M. A woman you do not know is trying to get you to do something. You do not know what it is she wants you to do. If she would show you what to do, you would do it, but you cannot understand a word she is saying. It all sounds like a foreign language. All you can say is "But I don't want to fish."

Player #2: Caregiver

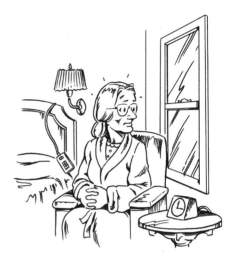

It is 8 A.M. Mrs. Jones has just finished breakfast. You want her to brush her teeth. She always has food stuck in her teeth and your supervisor is going to come back in 5 minutes to make sure her teeth are brushed. She is confused and you know you really need to work hard to get her to understand. Convince her to brush her teeth.

Situation #2

Mrs. James is 68 years old and lives in a nursing home. She has Alzheimer's disease and wanders everywhere. Right now she is walking out the front door of the home "for lunch," she says. It is actually 3 P.M. She insists that she really needs to hurry or she will be late. She is to "meet her sister at noon."

Player #1: Mrs. James

You must meet your sister at noon for lunch. You can only remember what the nursing assistant is telling you for about 30 seconds. Try to convince her that you need to leave, but the only thing you can say is "I'm meeting my sister for lunch. I have to meet her at noon."

Player #2: Caregiver

You see Mrs. James heading for the front door and she is telling everyone, "I'm meeting my sister for lunch. I have to meet her at noon." However, her sister died 3 years ago. It is winter and she is not wearing her coat and there is no one to go with her. Try to convince her not to go.

Figure 2.2.   Two role-playing situations for practicing communication techniques.

UNIT 2: QUIZ

Please take a few minutes to complete the quiz for this unit. Answer each question as best you can. Keep in mind this is a learning tool to help you summarize and remember what has been discussed in this unit. For true-false questions, check the correct answer. For multiple choice questions, circle the correct answer(s).

Note: There may be more than one correct answer for some questions.

1. When a person with dementia forgets the right word to use in a sentence, he or she also forgets the idea that he or she wanted to express.

    _____ True   _____ False

2. An effective communication technique when working with people with dementia is to remind them gently of past conversations.

    _____ True   _____ False

3. People with severe dementia are unable to understand emotional cues.

    _____ True   _____ False

4. All of the following communication mistakes may be found in people with mild dementia *except:*

    a. They will make frequent irrelevant comments.

    b. They will make repetitive movements, such as lip smacking.

    c. They are unable to recognize mistakes in speech.

    d. They will repeat the same word or phrase.

5. When communicating with someone who has dementia, all of the following should be done *except:*

    a. Touch the person gently.

    b. Obtain the undivided attention of the person.

    c. Use only one of the five senses to obtain the person's attention.

    d. Stand in the person's direct line of vision when speaking with him or her.

6. Mr. M., who is very forgetful, often misplaces items. You find Mr. M. very agitated because he has lost his watch. You should tell him that:

    a. He always misplaces things and should not be worried.

    b. You will help him look for it.

    c. You are busy right now but reassure him that he will eventually find it.

    d. The last time he lost his watch it was in the drawer and he should look for it there.

7. Mrs. A., who has dementia, is in the hall and very agitated. You should:

    a. Explain that there is no reason to be upset and you will walk her back to her room.

    b. Slowly take her hand and say, "I see that you are upset, may I help you?"

    c. Explain who you are and that she should go to the activities room and be with the others.

    d. Explain that her loud noise is disturbing the other residents and there is no reason to be upset.

8. The person who has severe dementia is unable to react to nonverbal communication cues such as a hug.

    ____ True   ____ False

UNIT 2: INSTRUCTOR HELP

1. Audiovisuals
   a. Portions of Table 2.1 are provided as transparencies in Appendix B. Review them with trainees, giving examples or explanations for each point, or ask the trainees to give examples of their own.
   b. The University of Washington videotapes on "Managing Aggressive Behaviors: Anger and Irritation, Catastrophic Reactions" (20 minutes) or "Managing Psychotic Behaviors: Language Deficits" (8 minutes) may be used. Preview them first and prepare an introductory explanation for the ones you show.

2. Discussion/questions
   a. Ask the trainees "How do we communicate?" Write down the answers on a blackboard and incorporate them into your presentation.
   b. Demonstrate, using body language, how the same words can be said repeatedly but send a different message each time. Be dramatic. After each demonstration, ask trainees to interpret. (Trainees can be asked to do these demonstrations.) The following is a list of some demonstrations that can be used:
      - Say "Good morning" while walking through the class. Use a monotone with no gestures.
      - Say "Good morning" as if the sun is shining and it is good to be alive. Have a brilliant smile and make quick eye contact, but do not touch anyone.
      - Say "Good morning" as if life is horrible. Make very brief eye contact.
      - Take a person's hand or touch his or her arm, then look him or her in the eye with a smile and say "Good morning."
      - Discuss the responses to each "Good morning" within the group.

3. Activities
   These activities are designed to sharpen trainees' awareness of how they communicate nonverbally and to underscore the importance of nonverbal communication. Train-

ees select partners and carry out each of the following exercises as directions are given.

- Standing 2 feet behind your partner, give directions for making coffee. When you are finished, have your partner repeat the directions as you have given. Repeat this exercise, but the second time, sit opposite your partner in a direct line of vision when you give directions. As a group, discuss how these experiences differ.

- Holding your partner's hand, ask how he or she feels right now. Switch roles and have your partner ask you the same thing but without holding hands. Discuss the impact of this kind of touching. Some participants may feel uncomfortable with touching, a feeling that may also be experienced by people with Alzheimer's disease. This may be personal, but it may also be tied to cultural convention. While touch is beneficial to the overwhelming majority of individuals, caregivers need to recognize when their efforts meet with displeasure.

- Direct one partner in each pair to role-play someone with Alzheimer's disease. Relying on nonverbal communication (gestures, facial expression, and voice tone), he or she should try to communicate a need (hungry, wet, thirsty, or warm). The individual may use one word, but that word must not mean what the person is trying to communicate. The partner should try to figure out the problem or the best response using simple statements, facial expressions, tone, and gestures.

The following are some strategies for improving verbal communication with people with Alzheimer's disease. Ask trainees to practice their communication in positive terms.

- Guide people with Alzheimer's disease to appropriate behavior by using positive language. State the following ideas in positive terms:

Do not put the ice cream in the stove.

Do not go over there.

You should not wear that coat when it is so hot outside.

You know that is not yours.

Do not move like that when I am trying to shave you.

- Avoid questions by stating ideas in positive terms. Turn the following questions into positive statements:

  What would you like to wear today?

  Who is the baby in this photograph?

  Do you want to wash up?

  Do you want to visit the doctor?

- Avoid applying reasoning and logic, instead, state what needs to be done. Offer an alternative response for the following statements that are not contradicting:

  You know that toothpaste goes on your teeth, not in your hair.

  Your sister died 3 years ago; she is not coming to visit you.

  Of course you know Mary. You worked with her for 25 years.

  You just asked me that question. You already know when your wife is coming.

You have been given several suggestions for activities that demonstrate communication. Of course, you cannot use them all during one session, but because communication is such a vital part of caring for people with Alzheimer's disease, it might be appropriate to try a short "communication activity" at the beginning or end of several sessions, particularly the ones on assisting with personal care. Each activity takes about 15–20 minutes, depending on the size of the class. Plan your time accordingly.

Appendix

I've Lost a Kingdom

A Victim's Remarks on Alzheimer's Disease

Articles on Alzheimer's disease appear everywhere. The disease is the major cause of death in the United States after heart disease, cancer, and stroke. Because the tragedy is common, because it is awesome, there cannot be too many articles on this topic. The possibility of reaping even a minuscule useful point from going over another report is enough to keep family members reading.

But what about the victims of the disease? How do they feel? People with cancer, heart disease, and stroke have written about their illnesses. Those with Alzheimer's disease, almost by definition, cannot. Marguerite R. Lerner, a successful physician and writer of children's books, had a brilliant record in college. In addition to many talents she had numerous interests—her family, all children, reading, writing, music, the theater, physical activities, and more. She had to stop working in her mid-fifties because of Alzheimer's disease. Her comments in this article are direct quotes recorded by her husband, Dr. Aaron B. Lerner. No editing was done. Most of the remarks were made in the period 1980–82 and were voiced in a calm manner between 3:00 and 5:00 A.M. Her thoughts were often fully lucid in the early morning.

> I have a neurological problem. Who needs it? No one.
>
> I can't tell you how terrible things have been for me—to go from health to nothing.
>
> Nobody likes me. I don't like myself either.

Lerner, A.B. (1984). I've lost a kingdom: A victim's remarks on Alzheimer's disease. *Journal of the American Geriatrics Society, 32*(12), 935; reprinted by permission.

I used to be a physician. I used to drive a car. What do I want? I don't want to be here.

I know that I am not functioning as a mother or a spouse. You have to do all the work.

Am I always going to be sick? It would be nice if someone could help me.

I don't sing anymore. I probably won't sing again.

The worst thing is not having anything to do. Nobody wants you. I can't take it.

I am afraid of everything.

I shouldn't be here. I am just waiting until I die.

I don't care about anything anymore.

All I do is nothing.

I don't have anything. I used to be a physician.

Look how nice these boys are—and what a terrible mother. How did I get this way? I must have taken a wrong turn.

I don't want to be here for another birthday.

You need a new wife. This one is no good anymore.

All I am is garbage. I belong in the garbage can.

I think that I am getting better and all the time I am getting worse.

The days go so slow for me.

I would rather be dead than what I am doing here because I am not doing anything.

No one knows my name anymore—because I am nothing.

I don't care whether or not I wake up.

I've lost everything—the Health Service, typing, and writing. I don't have any skills. All I do is eat. I have to go away. I can't read my own writing.

I am no good anymore. All that I do is to tell lies. I want to be cremated and have the ashes taken to Woods Hole.

I've had a good life—a successful marriage—good children—a good career. Now there is nothing for me. I've lived too long.

I used to be something.

It was so much fun with the students when I was a teacher.

It is hard when one becomes obsolete.

I've lost a kingdom.

When can I be dead? Soon I hope.

I wish I were a little girl again.

Unit 3

Managing Personal Care and Nutrition

Learning Objectives

1. To recognize the importance of accommodating past personal care habits of a person with Alzheimer's disease into current personal care routines

2. To identify behaviors in the person with Alzheimer's disease that may indicate certain needs (e.g., need for toileting)

3. To list two ways the environment can be changed to decrease confrontations when bathing or dressing a person with Alzheimer's disease

4. To describe two nutritional needs of people with Alzheimer's disease

Nursing care is aimed at keeping people healthy and safe. Comprehensive nursing care includes helping people with Alzheimer's disease maintain contact with other people and reality because human contact is central to being human. Comprehensive care is accomplished by encouraging people with Alzheimer's disease to do as much as they can for as long as they can. Although it is sometimes easier and less time consuming for caregivers to do things, it is important to encourage people with Alzheimer's disease to be as independent as possible to help maintain their self-esteem.

GENERAL NURSING CARE PRINCIPLES

Caregivers should always offer positive reinforcement. If caregivers feed a person with Alzheimer's disease, they should praise him or her for eating well. If that person can feed him- or herself, then caregivers should express how much they appreciate this behavior, rather than getting upset because the person has made a mess. As part of the disease process, abilities of people with Alzheimer's disease to follow directions and use good judgment deteriorate over time. Special care is needed to compensate for the loss of these abilities; however, no matter how good care is, abilities will still deteriorate. People's lives will be better and more comfortable with good care, even though the disease cannot be cured.

It is imperative that caregivers concentrate on what the person with Alzheimer's disease *can* do, not what he or she cannot do. For example, he or she may not be able to cut meat and feed him- or herself, but he or she can pick up toast and eat it independently. Caregivers need to change their own behaviors and responses to accommodate each person they assist. They should anticipate problems and plan how to avoid them.

Place pictures of the person's family in his or her room. This can encourage discussion. Pictures should be of relatives as they were in past years, not as they are now. People with Alzheimer's disease remember things as they were in the past.

Keep caregiving routines very structured. A regular routine creates no surprises and no new situations that require adaptation on the part of the person with Alzheimer's disease. This decreases confrontational and negative behaviors and makes everyone's day flow much more smoothly. Follow the personal care activities guide for quick hints on caring for people with Alzheimer's disease (see Table 3.1).

A key point to remember is that people with Alzheimer's disease love to laugh. They do not always know what they are laughing about, but the sheer pleasure of laughter is calming.

BATHING

Bath time can be a very pleasant experience for both the caregiver and the person with Alzheimer's disease or it can become a dreaded, confrontational time. This section discusses the physical, emotional, and environmental reasons that people with Alzheimer's disease may react negatively to bathing. If caregivers consider these issues and address them utilizing some of the suggested coping strategies, bath time can be a pos-

Table 3.1.   Personal care activities guide

GUIDELINES FOR MANAGING PERSONAL CARE

- Personal care offers opportunities for human interaction, enhancement of communication, and practice of social, mental, and physical skills.
- Activities should be structured for simplicity and consistency.
- Personal care activities are not absolutes; that is, an opportunity can be refused.
- Personal care activities are personal and should be performed in ways that will retain the dignity of the person with Alzheimer's disease and the care provider.

Toileting

- Mark the bathroom or bathroom door.
- Make sure the bathroom is accessible.
- Learn the person's usual urination and defecation schedule.
- Watch for signs of agitation, restlessness, or pulling at clothing that may indicate a need to urinate or defecate.
- Assist with removing clothing and getting the person into the correct position, if needed.
- Provide verbal cues if the person does not seem to understand what to do.

Bathing

- Try to adjust the bathing schedule to the person's prior habits.
- Consider the cultural background of the person in relation to bathing.
- Avoid discussing whether the bath is needed; simply continue with the activity, one step at a time. You cannot argue logically with a person with Alzheimer's disease.
- If the person is severely agitated, seems angry or frightened, stop the procedure and try again later.
- Never leave the person unattended in bath or shower.
- Talk the person through each step. Support efforts at self-care by helping him or her start the activity.

Dressing

- Decrease the number of choices the person has to make.
- Lay out clothing items in the order they should be put on.
- Replace buckles, buttons, zippers, and so forth with Velcro fasteners.
- Clothing that fastens in back may be useful for people who are incontinent or use a wheelchair, and for those who insist on removing their clothing.

GUIDELINES FOR MANAGING NUTRITION

Feeding

- Create as normal an eating situation as possible.
- Keep the experience positive by playing soft music in the background, giving the person adequate time to eat, and serving favorite foods.
- Offer a balanced diet.
- Be sure mouth care of some kind is performed at least twice a day.
- Consider prior eating habits, such as timing of meals and food preferences.

itive experience for all. Some physical and medical causes for negative reactions to bathing include the following:

- Depression or lack of interest
- Physical illness
- Altered sense of perception of hot and cold water temperature (as a result of damage in the hypothalamus region of the brain that regulates the "internal thermostat")
- Sensation of water is altered due to brain injury

Some altered cognitive and emotional causes for negative reactions to bathing include the following:

- Fear of falling
- Fear of water or being hurt by it
- Disruption in daily routine or schedule
- Fear of unfamiliar caregivers
- Being too overwhelmed by the mechanics of taking a bath
- Inability to remember the purpose of bathing
- Humiliation of being reminded to take a bath
- Agitation from an upsetting situation (e.g., an argument with caregiver)
- Feeling of being rushed by caregiver
- Feeling embarrassed and vulnerable about being naked or having another person in the bathroom
- Preference for same-sex caregiver, but inability to say so
- Fatigue
- Fear of getting hair washed because the purpose is no longer understood
- Impatience due to having waited too long while the caregiver prepares bath
- Fear of soap, washcloth, sound of running water, and so forth

Some environmental causes for negative reactions to bathing include the following:

- Dim lighting (The person may be unable to see the tub or shower, particularly if vision is also impaired and the person's glasses have been removed in preparation for bathing.)
- Lack of privacy
- Room that is too cold

- Water that is too deep
- Water that is too hot or cold

Coping Strategies for Caregivers

No single strategy for coping with people with Alzheimer's disease will work for every person with the disease. There are many strategies and at first it may take some time to see which ones will work for both the caregiver and the person with Alzheimer's disease. The following is a list of suggestions that may help:

- Try to be consistent with the person's old bathing routine, including time of day. If the person with Alzheimer's disease is still capable of making choices and would like to have a bath at another time than the time the caregiver selects, give the person a choice between two times during the day, and then be sure that the agreement is honored by the caregiver. For people with Alzheimer's disease who are still capable of exercising some control over their lives, it is important to give them opportunities to do so. Choice of bath time can be an important opportunity to some.

- Be sure the bathroom is warm enough.

- Close doors and curtains to provide privacy. Make sure that other caregivers respect the closed doors. Sometimes people forget.

- Provide adequate lighting in the bathroom, especially during evening hours.

- Prepare bath, soap, clothes, and other supplies ahead of time so the person will not have to wait. Planning ahead also prevents the bath water from getting cold.

- Use a quiet, calm approach when giving instructions (e.g., "Your bath is ready now."). If a person says, "I don't want to take a bath," quietly ignore the statement and slowly repeat the directions, then go on to the next step. This may divert his or her attention.

- Establish a routine. Do everything exactly the same way each time. If it is not possible to have the same caregiver every time a bath is needed, try very hard to find ways to convey the routine to other caregivers who may become involved.

- Check the temperature of water. The person's sense of temperature may be affected.

- Give the person a washcloth to hold as a distraction or to imitate the caregiver's washing motions.
- Wrap a towel around the shoulders of a person in the tub if he or she is embarrassed about being undressed. The towel wrap also helps to prevent chilling.
- Play soft music in the background; it can create a calming and relaxing atmosphere.

Safety Considerations for Bathing

Sometimes people with Alzheimer's disease are very fearful about bathing for reasons that they cannot express. They may have had a bad experience in the past or fallen in the tub. There may be altered sensory perception and cognitive changes that prevent them from recognizing the bathing equipment or understanding the procedure. Using a quiet, calm voice or soft music can help alleviate unexpressed fear. The following is a list of safety precautions caregivers should follow when bathing people with Alzheimer's disease:

- Be sure the water temperature is a safe 120°–130° F.
- Do not leave the person alone in the shower or bath even for a second.
- Use a nonslip bathmat. Be sure there are no puddles on the floor.
- Let the water drain out of the tub first if the patient is afraid of falling.
- Be careful about the slippery residue left in the tub if bath oil is used.
- Be sure that the area around the tub or shower is free from electrical appliances, such as radios and hair dryers, that could be pulled into the water. It is always best to unplug all bathroom electrical items during bath time.

Figure 3.1 is a reference sheet for determining the reasons for negative reactions to bathing and suggestions for appropriate action.

DRESSING

As with bathing, dressing is a task in which the caregiver of a person with Alzheimer's disease can encourage the person to make use of abilities that still exist. The person can be encour-

Keeping the Alzheimer patient clean and well-groomed can be a challenge for the caregiver. A depressed person might have lost her desire to bathe while another person might feel embarrassed about getting undressed or might become frightened by running water or mirrors.

For the person who has Alzheimer's, it's easy to feel confused and overwhelmed by simple daily routines such as bathing and grooming. If the person seems afraid, stressed or resistant to bathing, try to determine the reasons why by asking the following questions:

PHYSICAL/PSYCHOLOGICAL FACTORS

Does the person seem depressed?

- Is there a physical illness or infection?
- Does the person seem overly sensitive to water or changes in water temperature?

ENVIRONMENTAL FACTORS

Is the person sensitive about having someone else in the bathroom?

- Is the person able to find the bathroom and see clearly once she enters it?
- Is the room temperature too cold?
- Is the water temperature too hot or cold? Or is the water pressure too intense? Is the water in the tub too deep?

SPECIAL CONCERNS

Is the person afraid of falling, running water or soap? Or is the person confused over such tasks as turning on the water or filling the sink?

Once you've determined the answers to these questions, you'll be in a better position to manage the bathing routine.

ACTION STEPS

Have Reasonable Expectations

Keep in mind that frequency of washing and bathing is a personal preference. Some people may not feel the need to shower and/or wash their hair every day. In these cases you might want to alternate a sponge bath with a more complete bath or shower.

Adapt to the Patient's Needs, Routines, and Preferences

If the person is used to taking a shower in the morning or a bath at night, try to maintain that routine. Changing from day to night might distress the person. Also keep in mind that a person may refuse to take a bath for an unfamiliar caregiver of the opposite sex.

(continued)

Figure 3.1.   Guidelines for bathing. (From Alzheimer's Disease and Related Disorders Association, Inc. [1990]. *Bathing.* Chicago: Author; reprinted by permission.)

Figure 3.1 *(continued)*

Prepare the Bathroom in Advance

- Have the towels ready.
- Draw the water in the bathtub and test the temperature.
- Pre-measure the shampoo.
- Develop a soap pocket in the washcloth so that the person can wash herself.
- Keep the bathroom warm and comfortable.

Gently Prepare the Patient for the Bath

Be directive at bathtime by using such phrases as, "Your bath is ready." In this way, the person will focus on each step of the task instead of whether or not she needs or wants a bath. If the individual continues to resist the idea of bathing, distract her for a few moments and then try again.

Make the Bathroom Safe

- Always check the temperature of the water. Keep in mind that the person may not be able to judge temperature.
- Avoid using bubble bath or bath and shower oils that would make the tub or shower stall slippery.
- Keep in mind that showers are often more dangerous and frightening to people with Alzheimer's disease than baths. If you must use a shower, install grab bars and use a tub seat.

aged to make a choice between two dresses or two sweaters. If the clothes can be laid out on the bed in the order they are to be put on (e.g., dress on the bottom, underwear on top), many people with Alzheimer's disease can function well enough to put on the clothing with minimal assistance. Do not encourage the person to make clothing choices if he or she becomes frustrated or upset. Try to allow enough time for the person to do as much for him- or herself as possible. Some physical and medical causes for negative reactions to dressing include the following:

- Depression
- Physical illness
- Impaired vision
- Changes in gross motor skills (e.g., unsteady balance, problems with walking)
- Changes in fine motor coordination skills (e.g., difficulty with fastening buttons or closing a zipper)
- Memory loss (e.g., sometimes people with dementia no longer have the ability to remember if they are getting dressed or undressed, they may forget to change their clothes)

- Side effects of medications (e.g., antidepressants or antihypertensives, which may cause dizziness)
- Stiff joints that make it hard to raise arms above the head or bend the knees

Some altered cognitive and emotional causes for negative reactions to dressing include the following:

- Task that is too complicated
- Unclear instructions
- Inability to make decisions about what to wear
- Lack of understanding about how to get dressed
- Feeling of being rushed by a caregiver
- Fatigue
- Fear or anxiety
- Embarrassment about having to dress in front of the caregiver (This can be especially true if the person with Alzheimer's disease and the caregiver are of different sexes.)
- Humiliation of being reminded to get dressed
- Inability to recognize parts of the body

Some environmental causes for negative reactions to dressing include the following:

- Dim lighting
- Distractions (e.g., noise, people, clutter in room)
- Lack of privacy
- Room that is too cold

Coping Strategies for Caregivers

Caregivers need to be especially attentive to people with Alzheimer's disease when helping them dress. The following is a list of suggestions that may help:

- Have a good medical workup done on the person to discover any possible causes or medications that might contribute to problems with dressing.
- Have vision and eyeglasses checked.
- Have an evaluation for depression, particularly if the person is frequently unwilling to get up or get dressed in the morning.

- Show the person the clothing he or she will be wearing that day.
- Be sure all clothing items are right side out. The caregiver may need to hand the person his or her clothing, one piece at a time, and give step-by-step directions for how to put on each item. It may be easier for the caregiver to dress the person, but that person needs to feel a sense of worth—a sense of knowing he or she can still help him- or herself.
- Keep morning routines as familiar to the person as possible, and avoid delays or interruptions.
- Make sure the room is warm enough.
- Provide adequate lighting.
- Close room door and curtains to provide privacy.
- Try to make the room as familiar to the person as possible.
- Encourage the person to select his or her own clothes but keep choices simple.
- Label dresser drawers, describing their contents. If the person with Alzheimer's disease has lost the ability to read written words, the caregiver can use pictures of the drawer contents instead.
- Replace more complex fasteners (e.g., buttons, buckles, zippers, hooks and eyes) with simpler devices, such as Velcro fasteners.

Special Considerations for Dressing

Caregivers should be considerate of the person's privacy needs for dressing and bathing and allow people to do as much for themselves as possible. Tasks should be broken down into simple and manageable steps. It is important for people with Alzheimer's disease to wear street clothes every day—this helps raise morale. Also, if the caregiver perceives the person to be "bedridden" or ill, expectations of what that person may still do for him- or herself will probably be minimal.

Some people with Alzheimer's disease tend to undress themselves frequently. This is embarrassing and inconvenient, but remember that they are no longer able to understand what is appropriate. Clothing that is difficult to remove, such as jumpsuits that fasten in the back, should be worn. Evaluate each situation to find out why the person is removing his or her clothes. The following questions may help:

Is the person dressed too warmly?

Does he or she need to go to the bathroom?

Is he or she tired and trying to get ready for bed?

Is he or she bored?

Some people with Alzheimer's disease put on many layers of clothing regardless of the weather. They may do this for different reasons. Some older women, having always worn long sleeves, are uncomfortable in short sleeves. Try substituting long-sleeve blouses and dresses or adding a sweater. Also, try putting away unsightly clothes that are worn often and substituting them with more appropriate items. Again, evaluate the situation before patiently removing extra clothes, knowing it may be necessary to repeat this many times. The following questions may help.

Is there any reason why the person should wear extra clothing?

Is it really too hot or is the extra clothing just embarrassing to the caregiver?

Figure 3.2 is a reference sheet for determining the reasons for negative reactions to dressing and suggestions for appropriate action.

GROOMING

Grooming activities include combing hair, shaving, cleaning glasses, cutting and filing fingernails and toenails, and applying makeup and perhaps some perfume or after-shave lotion. These aspects of personal care can generate the same negative responses that often accompany bathing and dressing, but can contribute greatly to the person's self-esteem. It is important to encourage and support caregiving staff and family members' efforts in providing grooming activities or persuading the person with Alzheimer's disease to perform these activities.

TOILETING

Toileting can be a very difficult part of giving care, but it is probably the easiest to improve. When people with Alzheimer's disease are wandering, they are often looking for the bathroom. The caregiver should take them to one; otherwise, the person

Physical appearance is important to everyone's sense of self-esteem. For the person with Alzheimer's disease, the simple act of putting on clothing can be frustrating. For this reason, you need to manage dressing difficulties one-by-one. There are many reasons why the person with Alzheimer's might have problems dressing, including the following:

PHYSICAL PROBLEMS

Does the person have problems with balance or with motor skills that are needed to fasten buttons or close zippers?

INTELLECTUAL PROBLEMS

Does the person remember how to dress?

- Does she recognize her clothes?
- Is she aware of the time of day or season of the year?

ENVIRONMENT

Is the person troubled by lack of privacy, a cold room, poor lighting, or loud noises?

OTHER CONCERNS

Are you pressuring the person to get dressed quickly?

- Are you giving the person clear step-by-step instructions on how to dress or does the task seem too complicated?
- Is the person embarrassed or humiliated by dressing in front of a non-family caregiver?

Once you've answered these questions, you'll be in a better position to help the person get dressed.

ACTION STEPS

Recognize the Importance of Clothing and Self-Esteem

Keep in mind that getting dressed and looking presentable are critical to a person's sense of well-being and self-esteem.

Make It Easy for the Patient to Make Clothing Selections

Lay out proper clothes for the person, including appropriate selections for warm and cool weather.

- If appropriate, give the person an opportunity to select favorite outfits or colors.
- If the person insists on wearing the same clothes every day, try to launder these clothes often or get duplicates of favorite outfits. You many need to temporarily distract the individual as you remove clothing for cleaning.
- You may want to remove excess clothing from the closet. Seeing many clothes can be overwhelming and upsetting to the person.

(continued)

Figure 3.2. Guidelines for dressing. (From Alzheimer's Disease and Related Disorders Association, Inc. [1990]. *Dressing.* Chicago: Author; reprinted by permission.)

Figure 3.2   *(continued)*

Choose Clothing That's Practical

Select fabrics that are lightweight and flexible and feel soft and comfortable on the person's skin.

- In general, choose clothing that's durable, washable and flame retardant.

Consider Experimenting with Various Types of Fasteners

Keep in mind that pressure tape or Velcro can be used as a substitute for buttons, snaps and hooks.

- Other devices include large-ring or loop-handled zippers or tape loops.
- Many caregivers turn to jogging suits that are washable, comfortable and have few fasteners.

Pay Attention to the Feet

To give the person's feet adequate support, encourage wearing regular shoes instead of slippers.

- Slip-on styles with elasticized inserts on the top are easy to put on and remove.
- Sneakers or shoes with crepe soles can help to prevent falls. Have an extra pair of shoes on hand in case the person's feet swell and keep the feet warm with loose-fitting, easy-to-wear socks.

Prepare for Dressing

Give easy-to-understand instructions and simple clothing selections so the person can dress herself for as long as possible.

- Lay out clothes in the order the person will put them on and then assist her through each step of the dressing process.

Dress for Ease and Convenience

Choose comfortable and loose-fitting clothing that's easy to put on and remove.

- Many caregivers find that cardigans or tops that fasten in front are more comfortable and easier to work with than pullovers.
- To avoid tripping and falling, make sure that clothing length is appropriate.

Adapt Regular Clothes to the Needs of the Patient

If the patient is confined to a wheelchair, you might adapt regular clothes to protect the patient's privacy and allow for greater comfort.

- Make sure that clothing is loose-fitting, especially at the waist and hips—and choose fabrics that are soft, stretchable and slick.

Adjust to the Problems of Incontinence

If incontinence is a problem for the person, make sure that clothing is easy to remove and care for.

- Although some caregivers purchase protective pads, you might also want to add an extra layer of protection to regular clothing by lining the backs of skirts or pants with terrycloth material.

Helping the Alzheimer patient with her grooming and dressing will allow her to maintain a sense of dignity and positive self-esteem. It's important to remember to let the person perform daily dressing routines for as long as possible.

may void on the floor, in a waste can, or in some other undesirable place. A picture of a commode or a special bright color on the bathroom door may help people with Alzheimer's disease remember where the bathroom is located.

All people with Alzheimer's disease should be taken to the bathroom every 2 hours while they are awake, after every meal, and before going to bed.

Coping Strategies for Caregivers

If the person awakens during the night, he or she will want to go to the bathroom. A night light will help illuminate the area where the bathroom is located. It will also lessen the confusion of awakening in a dark place and not knowing where he or she is. Try to keep rooms and floors free of clutter so no accidents occur. People with Alzheimer's disease should be taken to the bathroom when they awaken in the morning. They may be stimulated to void immediately if their bare feet hit the cold floor. Even if they say they do not need to use the bathroom, they should have their underwear pulled down and be seated on the toilet. Running water in the bathroom may initiate the urge to void. Giving them a glass of water to drink also helps. Women can be more independent if they wear slacks with elastic waistbands. Men may benefit from a Velcro closing rather than a button on their slacks. Praise the person for everything he or she does correctly. Compassion and a sense of humor are essential!

If a person with Alzheimer's disease who formerly has been continent suddenly becomes incontinent, he or she needs to be evaluated for a possible urinary tract infection. Another possible cause of the incontinence is that a new medication such as a diuretic may have been started. If the latter is the case, the person will probably require more frequent toileting. Keep in mind that being in bed with siderails, being restrained, or lying on protective pads may give the person the idea that he or she is expected to be incontinent.

Be sure that a person with Alzheimer's disease is receiving enough fluids. He or she may not be aware of thirst. A good amount to give is 1½–2 quarts of fluid daily. This may include fruit juices and noncaffeinated beverages. Try to minimize caffeinated beverages, because caffeine is a diuretic and can contribute to incontinence.

Remember that the privacy considerations discussed in reference to bathing also apply to toileting.

EATING

Food is more than just nourishment for the body. From a human's first experience with it, food is associated with caring and nurturing. People with Alzheimer's disease still have these memories and associations of food; these are not lost with other memories.

People with Alzheimer's disease who are physically active or hyperactive burn large numbers of calories daily. In order for them to remain physically well, they must take in sufficient amounts of protein, calories, and fluids. This helps prevent skin breakdown and constipation and enhances the immune system. Food also contributes to general well-being.

During the last stages of Alzheimer's disease the body does not seem to utilize the calories that are eaten and the person often loses weight, regardless of intake, and becomes emaciated. This can be a very upsetting time for a caregiver if he or she does not understand the normal progression of Alzheimer's disease. Some physical and medical causes for negative reactions to eating include the following:

- Mouth discomfort from gum disease or ill-fitting dentures; dry mouth
- Vision change, causing inability to see food or utensils well
- Acute or chronic illness causing loss of appetite
- Constipation or depression causing loss of appetite
- Sense of taste altered from aging or medications
- Muscles of jaw or throat that no longer work properly because of motor decline in advanced dementia
- Inability to understand hunger sensations from the stomach or to receive hunger messages by the brain
- Inability to remember to stop and eat
- Reversal of day and night sleep patterns
- Side effects of medications (e.g., antidepressants)
- Agitation

Some altered cognitive and emotional causes for negative reactions to eating include the following:

- Inability to understand how to eat
- Inability to coordinate use of silverware
- Unclear or complicated instructions

- Feelings of being rushed by caregiver
- Caregiver's tension or impatience
- Fear or anxiety

Some environmental causes for negative reactions to eating include the following:

- Relocation to new environment
- Dim lighting
- Distraction (e.g., noise, people, too much food on plate)
- Boredom, which may cause desire to eat all the time
- Food that looks or smells unappetizing
- Odors in the dining room (e.g., urine, cleaning fluids)

Coping Strategies for Caregivers

Make sure people with Alzheimer's disease receive a thorough medical workup to discover any possible physical causes or medication problems that could be contributing to appetite change. Also, see that they have a good dental and vision check-up and are evaluated for depression. Eliminating physical causes for appetite change will help caregivers focus on the environmental causes.

Try to reduce noise and distractions in the dining area during meals by providing for small group dining. By using textured wall hangings, excessive noise can be reduced. Play soft, relaxing music during the meal. This may help people focus their attention on the enjoyment of eating. Also, reduce unpleasant odors and improve lighting around the tables, but avoid glare. Group people with Alzheimer's disease according to eating abilities, allowing particularly agitated individuals to eat alone. This should help ensure an uninterrupted meal for others.

Reduce distractions at the table by avoiding patterned place mats, plates, and tablecloths. Serve only one food at a time, if necessary, and remove other distracting items from the table.

Try to make eating simple. Use bowls and cups that are larger than the portion of food served and bowls or plates that are different in color from the place mat to help the person locate the plate more easily. Generally, try to use bowls rather than plates. This will help keep food from spilling out. If you use a plate, place a damp washcloth under it to keep it from sliding. Set place setting only with utensils that are needed for that meal. Do not use plastic utensils, which are too light to manipulate easily and may break in the person's mouth. For liquids, try bendable straws or cups with lids and spouts to prevent spillage. Use mugs for soups or stews and be sure handles are big enough for easy holding. For people who always have problems eating, use assistive devices such as large handled silverware, plates with rims, and so forth. Serve lots of finger foods that can be easily handled by all people with Alzheimer's disease (e.g., French fries, cheese cubes, small sandwiches, chicken or beef kebabs, fried chicken, fresh fruit, vegetable pieces). This will help people who have difficulty using utensils. Put a bite of food to the person's lips as a stimulus to open the mouth.

If a person with Alzheimer's disease has difficulty chewing, make sure the person is in a comfortable position and apply light pressure on the lips or under the chin to get chewing started. To further help stimulate a person to chew his or her food, demonstrate chewing and give verbal instructions (e.g., "Chew now. Now swallow."). Avoid foods that may stick to the roof of the mouth (e.g., bananas, peanut butter, white bread) and foods that fall apart or have tough skins (e.g., nuts). It may help to moisten food with sauces, gravy, or water. Some people have dry mouths from medications and this may cause problems swallowing.

Make sure food is offered in small bites, one at a time. Keep in mind that swallowing problems are very common in people with Alzheimer's disease, and aspiration of food particles and choking problems with liquids can easily occur. The following are some helpful measures:

• Remind the person to swallow with each bite.

• Stroke the throat gently downward.

• Check the mouth periodically for food that may be stored in a cheek.

• Avoid foods that are hard to chew and swallow.

• Allow plenty of time between each bite. A bite of food should be swallowed completely before the next bite is taken.

• Keep liquids at room temperature.

• Moisten foods.

• Try thick liquids.

• Add milk or water to cooked cereal.

If choking is a constant problem with solid foods, try soft cooked foods such as scrambled eggs, canned fruit, cottage cheese, frozen yogurt, Jell-O made with orange juice, chopped chicken, mashed potatoes, and applesauce.

If people with Alzheimer's disease have sweet cravings, check their medications first. Some antidepressants cause a craving for sweets. Gum may be offered if the person will chew it and not swallow it. Nutritious milk shakes or egg nogs can also help alleviate the craving for sweets.

For overeating or insatiable hunger, try offering five or six small meals a day. Have a tray of low-calorie snacks available. Sometimes the person can be distracted with activities, walks, or other exercise. If undereating is a problem, offer a glass of juice, wine, or sherry (if medications permit) before a meal to whet appetite. Try to serve favorite foods whenever possible, and offer treats such as ice cream or milk shakes, or mix puddings with other foods to sweeten.

Give supplements, such as Instant Breakfast, Sustacal, Ensure, or vitamin supplements. There are liquid forms available if swallowing pills is a problem. Try feeding all or most of one food before moving on to the next. Some people become confused when the tastes and textures change rapidly. Sit directly in front of the person if his or her peripheral vision is not good. Show each spoonful to help orient eating. Allow the person to eat when he or she is hungry, and make sure the person is getting enough exercise to stimulate an appetite.

Make sure meals are offered at regular, consistent times every day. Make mealtimes simple and relaxed, and allow enough time for the person to eat. Feeding people with Alzheimer's disease in the last stages may take 45 minutes to an hour. Be sure the person is in a comfortable, upright position for eating. If necessary, coordinate tranquilizing medications with mealtimes to reduce agitation, and verbally guide the person through the meal, if necessary, using simple, gentle, respectful language. This should help make mealtime more pleasant. Consider the use of aprons instead of towels or gowns to protect clothing during meals. Also, try making milk, coffee, or juice available first thing in the morning to take the edge off morning hunger.

Everyone who assists with feeding people with Alzheimer's disease should follow these tips:

• Allow enough time for each bite.

• Use verbal cues and reminders.

• Allow people to feed themselves whenever possible.

• Gently wipe the person's mouth between bites.

- Concentrate on the person being fed. Do not talk or socialize with other staff.

- Encourage those staff members who have been successful in feeding someone difficult to feed that person consistently whenever possible.

Special Considerations for Eating

Observe carefully to assess what might be causing an eating or feeding problem. Is the problem with use of silverware, chewing, swallowing, distraction, noise, too much food on the plate, or is the caregiver too impatient? Keep in mind the person's past history with food. He or she always may have had a small appetite, been a voracious eater, or had a craving for sweets. Some eating problems are temporary and will eventually pass as the person's abilities change. Pay close attention to food temperature. Even though warm food is more appetizing, some people may have lost the ability to judge when food or drink is too hot. For this reason, use of styrofoam cups is not recommended because they hold the heat for a long time. Other disadvantages of using styrofoam cups are that they tip over easily and some people try to eat the styrofoam.

Many people with Alzheimer's disease do not get enough liquids because they have lost their sense of thirst. Offer regular drinks of water, juice, or other fluids to avoid dehydration. Also remember that mouth care is extremely important for people with Alzheimer's disease. Teeth need to be brushed at least twice a day.

Some people with Alzheimer's disease reach a point where they are unable to swallow or they simply refuse to eat. It is important for families to discuss feelings ahead of time about the use of feeding tubes. To use or not to use a feeding tube is a very personal, individual decision, but one that needs to be made in advance and discussed with medical personnel.

Figures 3.3 and 3.4 are reference sheets for assessing problems in eating and maintaining proper nutrition. Each figure also suggests appropriate actions for the caregiver.

Many Alzheimer patients have problems with eating. For example, a person might lose his appetite or the ability to evaluate if food is too hot or too cold. In addition, a person might forget that he's eaten and ask you for another meal. Begin by assessing the problem. Ask yourself: "Why is the person having difficulty eating?" The following questions are helpful:

PHYSICAL DIFFICULTIES

Is the problem physical? Sores in the mouth, poor-fitting dentures, gum disease, or dry mouth may make eating difficult. A visit to your physician might be helpful.

DISEASE

Does the person have an additional chronic disease? Intestinal or cardiac problems or diabetes might lead to loss of appetite. Constipation or depression can also decrease appetite.

AGITATION/DISTRACTION

Is the person agitated or distracted? If agitated, the person probably won't sit still long enough to eat an entire meal. If the person is distracted, you might want to think about how you can reduce distractions in the room.

EATING STYLE

Have you recently changed eating styles? Does the person have a preferred eating style? Some Alzheimer patients who aren't accustomed to sitting down at the table for three full meals may prefer to have several smaller meals or snacks.

VISUAL PROBLEMS

Can the person see adequately? An Alzheimer patient who had been losing weight began to eat when she started wearing her glasses at mealtimes.

ENVIRONMENT

Are there odors or harsh noises in the room that might interfere with the person's digestion?

FOOD QUALITY

Is the food appealing—in appearance, smell and taste? Once you've evaluated the sources of eating problems, you can take action.

ACTION STEPS

Adapt to the Person's Food Preferences

Remember that you're dealing with a person who has long-standing personal preferences and tastes. Try to keep these likes and dislikes in mind when you're preparing food. On the other hand, the person may no longer remember her favorite foods.

(continued)

Figure 3.3.   Guidelines for eating. (From Alzheimer's Disease and Related Disorders Association, Inc. [1990]. *Eating.* Chicago: Author; reprinted by permission.)

Figure 3.3   *(continued)*

Try to Reduce Mealtime Confusion

- Provide a calm environment at mealtimes. Minimize distractions, loud noises, and abrupt movements.
- Offer meals at regular times.
- Make mealtime a pleasant but simple event. For example, put only one item of food on the plate at a time.
- Give the person only one utensil at a time. You may want to omit the knife from the place setting. Avoid using plastic utensils because they may break.
- Avoid patterned plates, tablecloths and placemats that might confuse and distract the patient. In most cases, use plain white plates or bowls and a contrasting placemat.
- Deliver simple, easy-to-understand instructions. For example, "Pick up your fork. Put some food on it. Raise it to your mouth."
- Be patient. Don't criticize the person's eating habits or urge him to eat faster.
- Speak slowly and clearly. Be consistent and repeat instructions in the same words each time.
- Be realistic about going out to eat. Avoid noisy or large restaurants and choose those that are small, comfortable, and familiar. Only you can decide if the person can order directly from the menu. As an alternative, you might want to order for the person.
- Make positive use of distractions. If the person resists eating, take a break, involve her in another activity, and return to eating later.
- Use memory aids to remind the person about meal times. You might try a clock with large numbers, an easy-to-read appointment calendar with large letters and numbers, or a chalk bulletin board for recording the daily schedule.

Minimize Problems in Chewing and Swallowing

Avoid foods such as nuts, popcorn, and raw carrots which may get lodged in the throat. Instead grind foods or cut them into bite-size pieces. Pureed and frozen foods can be stored in plastic bags for later use.

- Gently explain that the person should chew the food, eat slowly, and swallow.
- Encourage the person to sit up straight with her head slightly forward. If the person's head tilts backward, move it to a forward position.
- Serve soft foods such as applesauce, cottage cheese, and scrambled eggs.
- Serve thicker liquids such as shakes, nectars, and thick juices or serve a liquid along with the food.
- Learn the Heimlich maneuver in order to help the person if choking occurs.

Experiment with Solutions to Decrease Appetite

- Serve a glass of juice before the meal to stimulate the appetite.
- Prepare some of the person's favorite foods.
- Increase the person's physical activity.
- Plan for several small meals rather than three large meals.
- Give the person plenty to drink—especially in warm weather.
- Consider the use of food supplements such as instant breakfast, eggnog mixes, yogurt, and milk shakes.

(continued)

Figure 3.3   *(continued)*

Assist the Person to Function Independently

- Serve finger foods or serve the meal in the form of a sandwich.
- Serve food in large bowls instead of plates or use plates with rims or protective edges.
- Use spoons with large handles instead of forks.
- Set bowls and plates on a non-skid surface such as a cloth or towel.
- Use cups and mugs with lids to prevent spilling and fill glasses half full: use straws that bend.
- Use plastic tablecloths, napkins, or aprons to make cleanups easier.
- Gently place the person's hand on or near an eating utensil.
- Show the person how to eat by demonstrating eating behavior or by doing hand-in-hand feeding. After you get the first bite of food to the mouth, the person will often begin to eat.
- Give the person plenty of time to eat. Keep in mind that it can take an hour or more to feed a patient.
- Give the person the opportunity to eat with other family members for as long as possible.

Work to Prevent Eating and Nutrition Problems

- Use vitamin supplements only on the recommendation of a physician. Monitor their use.
- Don't serve steaming or extremely hot foods or liquids. Remember, the person might not be able to tell if the food or beverage is too hot to eat or drink.
- Limit or eliminate highly salted foods or sweets if the patient has a chronic health problem such as diabetes or hypertension.
- Control potential weight gains. If the person always seems hungry, serve smaller portions of food at more frequent intervals. Fill the gaps between regular meals with healthy snacks.
- After the meal is over, check to see that the person swallowed the food and nothing remains in the mouth.
- Restrict portions when appropriate. A person with Alzheimer's may have no concept of how much she's eaten.
- Keep in mind that the person may not remember when or if she ate. If the individual continues to ask about eating breakfast, you might consider serving several breakfasts—juice, followed by toast, followed by cereal.
- Help the person maintain good oral hygiene. If it's difficult to use a toothbrush, try oral swabs. Keep in mind that regular visits to the dentist are important.

Providing the Alzheimer patient with nutritious meals and snacks is a problem for many caregivers. Often the patient can't sense or identify hunger or fullness or the need for fluids or foods with certain vitamins and minerals.

PREDICTABILITY

The person's response to food is also difficult to predict. An individual might like specific foods such as turkey or chicken and then—without warning—turn away from these foods.

POOR NUTRITION

The result of poor nutrition among Alzheimer patients is usually weight loss or gain and a variety of other symptoms, including poor-fitting dentures, listlessness, and fatigue.

- A person who snacks regularly on such foods as candy and pastries often experiences a "sugar high" followed by complaints of being tired, depressed, or hungry.
- "Junk foods" tend to make the person more restless and disoriented and reduce the craving for regular meals and more nutritious foods.
- The person may also experience bowel or bladder problems because of not drinking enough fluids or eating adequate fiber.

DISEASE PROGRESSION

As the disease progresses, providing the person with proper nutrition may become even more difficult.

- The individual might not understand the timing of meals or the difference between breakfast, lunch, dinner, and snacks.
- In addition, you may have to offer more coaching at mealtime to help the person use utensils for chewing, swallowing, or identifying various foods. For example, you may hand the person a spoon only to discover that he can't remember how to use it.
- In another situation, a person who feels no need for food may clench his jaw tightly and refuse to let you put a utensil near his mouth. This person may not understand or remember what to do with food.

ACTION STEPS

Watch Out for Danger Signs and Take Action

Look for early behavior changes such as increased snacking, drastic shifts in food likes and dislikes, dramatic weight losses or gains, or bowel problems. Experiment with changes in the person's diet to address these problems. You may need to allow for more time and offer more assistance at mealtime.

Monitor Changes

Check the person's weight weekly and, on the advice of your doctor, have regular blood work completed, as needed. Laboratory reports will help to identify problems with cholesterol, anemia, dehydration, or constipation.

(continued)

Figure 3.4.   Guidelines for nutrition. (From Alzheimer's Disease and Related Disorders Association, Inc. [1990]. *Nutrition.* Chicago: Author; reprinted by permission.)

Figure 3.4   *(continued)*

Prepare Foods for Easier Chewing

If the person has problems with chewing, swallowing, or choking, try chopping or cutting the food into bite-size pieces.

Use Food to Trigger the Patient's Attention

Use rough-textured foods such as toast or sandwiches made on toasted bread to stimulate the person's tongue and encourage chewing and swallowing.

- The person with Alzheimer's sometimes has little sensation of food in the mouth. By gently moving the person's chin, you can remind him to chew.
- Stimulate chewing by touching the person's tongue with a fork or spoon. By lightly stroking his throat, you can remind him to swallow.

Use Soft Foods to Assist the Person

A person who has problems chewing or who has poor-fitting dentures will benefit from foods of soft textures such as a peanut butter sandwich rather than a sandwich made of sliced meat, or a mashed potato rather than a fried potato.

- You may want to serve mashed or steamed vegetables, bite-size pieces of cooked meat, or turkey or chicken salads instead of sliced meat.
- If swallowing becomes a problem, put food into a food processor or blender before serving it. Also remember that soups with two consistencies may confuse the individual.

Make Knife-and-Fork Foods into Finger Foods

If the person's regular breakfast consists of scrambled eggs and bacon, cut the food into small squares. Or combine cheese, meat, and eggs into an omelette so the person can pick up food with his fingers.

Proceed with Caution in Using Liquid Supplements

Liquid food supplements are often costly, high in sodium, and can sometimes be prepared more economically at home. If the person is eating regular meals, use supplements as an occasional between-meal or late-night snack or when the person refuses to eat a regularly scheduled meal. When considering supplements, consult with your physician.

Work to Make Mealtime Calm and Comfortable

Keep the environment quiet and free from such distractions as the television or radio.

- Try to maintain regular meals with the family for as long as possible. Social interaction and conversation are important.
- Feed the person at regular intervals. Many caregivers find it helpful to serve several small meals rather than three large meals.
- Be consistent. Feed the person in the same area at every meal and at the same approximate times each day.

(continued)

Figure 3.4 *(continued)*

- Keep the table setting simple. Avoid placing objects on the table that might distract or confuse the individual.
- Put condiments on food before serving it to the person.
- Set the table only with the utensils needed to eat the meal.
- Avoid using plates or placemats with patterns that might confuse the individual.
- Use a plate that's a different color from the placemat.
- Offer one food item at a time. A full plate with a meat, potato, and vegetable might overwhelm and confuse the person.
- Rely on nutritious finger foods as between meal supplements.
- Encourage independence for as long as possible by allowing the person to use utensils and eat finger foods. Holding a cup and drinking fluids through a straw will also give the person a sense of accomplishment.
- Serve thick fluids to prevent choking. If choking occurs, be prepared to use the abdominal thrust to dislodge the food.
- Prepare the meal ahead of time so you can stay with the person during the meal. He may mimic your eating behavior.
- Reduce between-meal snacks to ensure that the person eats at regular meals or provide the person with fruit or nutritious snacks.

UNIT 3: QUIZ

Please take a few minutes to complete the quiz for this unit. Answer each question as best you can. Keep in mind this is a learning tool to help you summarize and remember what has been discussed in this unit. For true-false questions, check the correct answer. For multiple choice questions, circle the correct answer(s).

Note: There may be more than one correct answer for some questions.

1. Which of the following techniques is *wrong* for working with a person who has difficulty eating?

   a. Mix all the food together.

   b. If a person is no longer able to use a fork or spoon, serve "finger foods."

   c. Limit the number of foods and utensils placed in front of a person.

   d. Allow the person to do as much for him- or herself as possible.

2. All of the following factors should be considered when planning or organizing personal care activities *except:*

   a. Keep personal care activities simple.

   b. Structure all personal care activities.

   c. Perform personal care activities only at allotted time.

   d. Supervise personal care activities.

3. Personal care activities can cause a catastrophic reaction because of the person's reluctance to share these activities with staff.

   ____ True   ____ False

4. It is more important to finish the baths assigned to you on a given shift than to take the time to let people "do it themselves" and not finish your assignment.

    ____ True   ____ False

5. All of the following techniques are helpful when bathing a person with Alzheimer's disease *except:*

    a. Avoid discussion of whether the bath is needed.

    b. Leave the person alone if he or she becomes agitated during the bath.

    c. Remember the person's cultural background and what bathing may mean to this person.

    d. Consider alternate ways of bathing, such as a sponge bath.

6. List three strategies to assist people who have trouble swallowing.

    a. _____

    b. _____

    c. _____

7. List three considerations that may make bath time more positive for the person with Alzheimer's disease.

    a. _____

    b. _____

    c. _____

8. All of the following techniques are useful when helping the person with Alzheimer's disease get dressed *except:*

   a. Simplify and structure the process.

   b. Eliminate accessories such as belts, ties, or scarves.

   c. Give a person many clothing items to choose from to exercise his or her "thinking" abilities.

   d. Put the clothes out in the order they are put on.

9. One very pleasant behavior that people with Alzheimer's disease usually do not lose is the ability to _____.

UNIT 3: INSTRUCTOR HELP

1. Audiovisuals

   a. Two transparencies from Table 3.1 are provided in Appendix B. Review the guidelines for managing personal care (toileting, bathing, dressing) and the guidelines for managing nutrition (feeding). You may wish to ask the trainees if these guidelines are practiced in their respective care facilities and homes.

   b. A videotape from the University of Washington on "Managing Personal Hygiene" (11 minutes) is helpful.

   c. You will need a blackboard, whiteboard, or something on which to write.

2. Discussion/questions

   There is a lot of content in this unit. You may wish to divide the class into two sessions.

   a. A good opening strategy is to ask trainees to list the progression of their own morning routine. Write comments on the blackboard. Then ask them if they bathe or shower in the morning or evening and why. Ask them if they brush their teeth before or after breakfast and why.

   b. Ask those who bathe in the evening, "What would you do if you suddenly were told you would have to take your bath at 9 A.M. each morning?

   c. Ask trainees to imagine that they are 80 years old and a 20-year-old "little girl" says to them, "Well, I can't help it. You must do it now." How would they feel? Point out that their reactions would be no different from those of people with Alzheimer's disease. Habits and attitudes are ingrained and may not be affected by the disease.

   d. After covering the content in each section, trainees might select a real resident from the facility and write a care plan for him or her utilizing what they have just learned.

   e. Some of the role-playing vignettes used in Unit 2 could be enacted again, particularly those that "persuade" a person with Alzheimer's disease to do something. This would help trainees develop words and phrases that are nonconfrontive.

Unit 4

Managing Difficult Behaviors

Wandering, Inappropriate Sexual Behavior, Anger, and Catastrophic Reactions

Learning Objectives

1. To identify three strategies for dealing with people with Alzheimer's disease who wander
2. To list three possible physiological causes of difficult behavior
3. To discuss the impact of the person's environment on his or her difficult behavior
4. To identify possible meanings behind a person's difficult behavior

There are many difficult behaviors the caregiver must be able to cope with and handle when caring for a person with Alzheimer's disease. Some of the problems that the caregiver may face include wandering behavior, inappropriate sexual behavior, and catastrophic reactions.

WANDERING BEHAVIOR

Wandering behavior does not occur continuously through the day but it may occur during any time of the day or night. This behavior is a problem for people with Alzheimer's disease and caregivers because of the potential for injury. Wandering can result in death from exposure to the elements. It is exhibited in more than 75% of people with Alzheimer's disease at some point during their disease process.

It can be very difficult to determine the cause of the wandering. Often, the behavior will suddenly cease for no reason that is apparent to the caregiver. Efforts to control wandering can result in a confrontational situation between the person and caregiver, which may cause the problem to escalate.

If the person with Alzheimer's disease is wandering, consider the possibility that he or she may need to go to the bathroom or that he or she may be hungry, thirsty, cold, or simply want a more comfortable bed. Perhaps the person needs a room with better light, or had always coped with stress by walking and needs to exercise. Reactions to medications, physical illness, and dehydration all contribute to confusion, thereby increasing the risk of wandering.

Sometimes the person may wander because he or she is seeking spatial understanding of his or her physical environment or searching for home or people from the past. He or she may be responding to previous work roles that required walking.

Social and emotional needs frequently cause the person with Alzheimer's disease to wander. He or she may feel bored, lonely, anxious, trapped, closed in, or fearful because a caregiver or family member is out of sight. The person may be sensing a caregiver's anger and trying to get away from it.

Nighttime wandering especially is difficult for caregivers. It prevents sound sleeping by the caregiver and causes fatigue, thus causing more stress. Some possible causes of nighttime wandering are the following:

- Inability to separate dreams from reality
- Inactivity or too much sleep during the day
- Adverse (paradoxical) reaction to tranquilizers or sleep medications
- Inability to differentiate day and night
- Disorientation to time (i.e., when a person wakes up, he or she thinks it is time to get up)

Determining the Risk of Wandering

Not all people with Alzheimer's disease are at high risk for wandering. It is possible to evaluate people to determine if they are at risk. They usually have sufficient cognitive impairments that contribute to getting lost, but also have sufficient social skills to somewhat mask these deficits. If an individual who exhibits wandering behavior is admitted to a care facility, this fact should be communicated to the caregiving staff at the time of admission. People who wander are likely to escape notice of the staff and, therefore, be at risk for leaving. People who wander may present some or all of the following characteristics:

• Increased speech and reading problems
• Incontinence
• Constant disorientation
• Inability to realize they are lost
• Good social skills
• Good hearing
• Mobility with good gait and tendency to be continuously active

Reasons People Wander

With help from the family of a person with wandering behavior, develop a social and medical history that includes information about the person's way of coping with change and stress, patterns of physical exercise, and lifetime habits both at work and home. This information may be helpful in determining whether the wandering is related to previous lifestyles. For example, a person who wanders at the same time every day may be returning to a former schedule or routine (e.g., trying to get back to work after lunch), or wandering may be the result of the person searching for a part of life lost to the disease. Sometimes, after a move into a care facility, it is not uncommon for a person to become disoriented when awakening in the middle of the night. Wanderers are often searching for a familiar person, place, or possession. Reminiscing about the past may be comforting, and help stop the wandering behavior.

Frequent wandering can be a coping mechanism to relieve stress and tension. Trying to stop the wandering behavior may increase agitation and cause anger and frustration for the person. A written log about the behavior may be helpful in understanding what leads to wandering (e.g., Is the person trying to find a room? What was going on before the wandering started? What time of day is it?). Also, monitor all medications, especially if antidepressants or antianxiety drugs recently have been changed or introduced. Keep this in a record, too.

Some useful techniques that may help prevent people from wandering include the following:

- Ask people who wander to sit in bean bag chairs. Bean bag chairs are harder to get in and out of than regular chairs.

- Have a plan of action in case someone wanders away from the care facility or from home. Make sure other caregivers are aware of the plan.

- Using medications such as Haldol and Mellaril may be helpful in controlling the agitation that leads to wandering, but they should be used only if wandering behavior is uncontrollable and causes injury. Some people may develop a paradoxical reaction and experience *increased* restlessness.

- Using physical restraints of any type are a last resort (i.e., when all other strategies have failed and the person is at risk of injuring him- or herself). They usually add to the stress and agitation of the wanderer.

Tips for designing a special care unit to minimize wandering are in Unit 7.

Figure 4.1 is a handy guide summarizing the key points to remember about wandering behavior. It offers suggestions to determine the reasons for wandering and interventions for the behavior.

Coping Strategies for Caregivers

Some strategies to use to help cope with people who wander include the following:

- Make sure the person has a thorough medical evaluation, particularly if wandering begins suddenly.

- Consider possible physical causes (e.g., illness, hunger).

- Allow the person to wander if the environment is safe and secure.

- Place familiar objects, furniture, or pictures in the person's surroundings.

- Help direct a person through clearly labeled rooms (e.g., door decorations or name plaques, picture of toilet on bathroom door).

- Decrease noise levels and the number of people interacting with a wanderer at one time.

There are many reasons why an Alzheimer patient wanders or walks away from home or a well-known path or area. As a first step, try to determine the reasons behind wandering by asking these questions:

MEDICATION

Some medications have side effects that result in confusion and restlessness. Is the patient on such medication? If so, consult your physician.

STRESS

Is the person trying to handle stress, noise, unpleasant people, crowding, or isolation? If so, consider changing the situation.

TIME CONFUSION

Does the person become confused at certain parts of the day, such as the middle of the night or early evening? Does the person claim that people have been gone for days or weeks and then searches for them?

BASIC NEEDS

Is the person looking for something specific such as food, drink, the bathroom, or companionship?

RESTLESSNESS

Does the person have enough movement and activity during the day? Is it possible that the person wanders in order to get up and move around?

LACK OF RECOGNITION

Is the person in a new or changed physical environment that makes him want to search for familiar objects, surroundings or people?

FEAR

Is the person trying to escape from something frightening? Is the person experiencing a delusion or hallucination, or has the person simply misinterpreted sights and sounds?

PAST BEHAVIOR

Is the person trying to meet former obligations involving a former job, home, friend, or family member?

Other factors that may contribute to wandering include medical conditions such as stroke or other factors such as consumption of alcohol, changes in the weather, or feeling abandoned, useless or helpless. Wandering may be frustrating and irritating for caregivers, but it becomes a problem only when the person moves into an unsafe or unhealthy area or climate, puts others at risk or invades others' property.

For this reason, many people who care for Alzheimer patients decide to overlook wandering behavior until it becomes dangerous to the patient and to others. Or they permit the person to wander within safe boundaries or follow the individual on special outings.

(continued)

Figure 4.1. Guidelines for wandering. (From Alzheimer's Disease and Related Disorders Association, Inc. [1990]. *Wandering.* Chicago: Author; reprinted by permission.)

Figure 4.1.   *(continued)*

ACTION STEPS

Be Prepared

Be aware that wandering may or may not happen. There's no way to predict who will wander or when and how it might happen. Some people never get lost and others get lost frequently. The best advice is to be prepared. If the person has a daily exercise routine and hasn't yet wandered, you needn't be overly concerned. However, once the person begins to wander or gets lost, you should watch him more closely.

Encourage Movement and Exercise

Allow the person to move within safe areas or make a shared exercise such as walking part of your daily routine. Although walking in a circle might seem unusual, keep in mind that physical activity—from walking and sweeping, to rolling yarn or folding clothes—is a positive experience for the person with Alzheimer's.

Be Objective

Don't take the person's wandering behavior personally. The individual is probably trying to make sense of a world that no longer seems predictable.

Be Aware of Hazards

Remember that places that look safe might be dangerous for the person with Alzheimer's. For this reason, you should review the environment around your home for possible hazards, such as fences and gates, bodies of water, swimming pools, dense foliage, tunnels, bus stops, steep stairways, high balconies, and roadways where traffic tends to be heavy.

Secure Your Living Area

Do whatever you can to keep your home safe and secure. Place locks out of the normal line of vision—either very high or very low on doors. In addition, use a double bolt door lock, keeping the key handy for emergencies. Also use a child proof door knob that prevents the person with Alzheimer's from opening the door. Other effective safety actions include the following:

- Put hedges or fences around your patio or yard.
- Place locks on gates.
- Consider electronic buzzers, infrared electronic eye alarms, or chimes on your doors.
- Place a pressure sensitive mat at the door or person's bedside.
- Camouflage some doors with a screen or curtain, or put a two-foot square of a dark color in front of the door knob.
- Use a recliner or rocking chair; the person may need assistance to get up.
- Use nightlights, signs, and familiar objects to help the person move around in a safe area.
- Put gates at dangerous stairwells.

Communicate with the Person

Remind the person that you know how to find him and that he's in the right place. If possible, take the person for rides in cars or buses in addition to providing regular activity and exercise. And continually reassure the person, who may feel lost or abandoned.

(continued)

Figure 4.1. *(continued)*

Involve Your Neighbors

Inform your neighbors of the person's condition and keep a list of their names and telephone numbers handy. Although neighbors can be helpful in guiding the person home, you'll probably want to teach them how to approach the person with Alzheimer's disease by using these steps:

- Approach the person from the front.
- Introduce yourself and call or ask a name.
- Gently look for or ask to see identification.
- Offer help and re-establish the day, date, and time.
- Avoid pulling or pushing the person.
- Report the patient found.

Involve the Police

Some police departments keep a photo and fingerprints of people with Alzheimer's on file. Many local Alzheimer's Association Chapters sponsor some kind of identification program to help with wandering patients. If a person with Alzheimer's becomes lost, take a photo and an article of unwashed, worn clothing in a plastic bag to the police. Also have data on the following items:

- Age
- Hair color
- Blood type
- Eye color

- Identifying marks
- Medical condition
- Medication
- Dental work

- Jewelry
- Allergies
- Complexion

Offer suggestions about where the police might find the patient, such as old neighborhoods, former workplaces, or favorite places.

Be Prepared for Other Modes of Wandering

Although most wandering takes place by foot, some individuals with Alzheimer's disease have been known to drive 300 miles—sometimes in an automobile that belongs to someone else. You can prevent these problems by keeping car keys out of sight or by temporarily disabling the car by removing its distributor cap.

SPECIAL RECOMMENDATIONS FOR LONG-TERM CARE FACILITIES

Use Medication with Caution

Keep in mind that no medication controls wandering. If medicated, some patients actually become more agitated. Other medications bring about complications related to immobility.

Respond to Wanderers as Individuals

Keep the patient busy in full view of the staff and help the patient develop a walking route around the facility.

Develop a Procedure for Handling Missing Residents

Be sure to include such steps as searching the facility, calling the administrator, and notifying a family member who will then notify the police. In some cases, the facility may need to notify the police.

Inform People About How to Approach a Patient

Invite policemen, firemen, business people, and family members to in-service workshops on how to help wanderers. Help them understand that wanderers should be approached calmly and then reassured and guided back to the facility.

- Encourage walking or exercise. Caregivers may have to accompany the person.
- Remove items from a person's surrounding that may trigger desire to go out (e.g., shoes, coat, purse).
- Distract the person with conversation, food, drink, or activity.
- Be sure that the person is not wandering because he or she needs to use the bathroom. Look for signals such as fidgeting with clothes. At night, a bathroom or commode should be readily available.

Other suggested solutions for managing people with wandering behavior or other difficult behaviors are in Table 4.1.

Communication techniques, appropriately applied, can sometimes alleviate or prevent wandering. It is important to remember that communication is the most important aspect of caring for the person with Alzheimer's disease. Patience and a sense of humor are other useful attributes for the caregiver. Some techniques that may be helpful in communicating with a person who wanders include the following:

- Reassure the person frequently about where he or she is and why.
- Speak in a calm, normal tone of voice.
- Try written assurance for a person with mild impairments to reinforce an anticipated event (e.g., a written note saying, "Jane will be here at 3 P.M.").
- Try not to confront or argue with the person who is wandering. This only leads to a "no win" situation. Limit the number of people who redirect a wanderer. If more than one person is needed for safety, the second person can remain out of sight or in the background behind the other caregiver.
- Increase the wanderer's trust by humoring and cajoling.
- Allow the person to verbalize without arguing.
- Alleviate fears.
- Approach the wanderer in a casual, nonthreatening manner. It is best to approach the wanderer slowly and calmly from the front. Fall into step beside him or her and walk a short distance with the person before gently guiding him or her back to the activity, event, or location.
- Give the wanderer verbal identification of person, place, and time.

Table 4.1. Suggested solutions for managing difficult behaviors

Situation	Suggested solutions
Person refuses to take a bath.	Offer a shower. Try a different caregiver. Do not get angry. Leave resident alone. Offer again later.
Person repeats, "I want to have 'choice' staff."	Try to interpret the meaning of the words. If you cannot, smile and hug the person.
Person says to his wife, "I want to see my wife."	Remember the person really believes he is not talking to his wife. Give support, not persuasion. Understand that his wife also needs support.
Person walks up to staff member and pinches him or her.	Walk away quietly. If behavior persists, put your hand over the person's and simply state, "Let go."
Person is walking out the front door and going "home for lunch."	Say, "Let's go together," and walk off in the same direction. Use the time to change the subject and slowly turn around. Feed the resident.
Person repeats the same question over and over.	Ignore him or her. He or she usually will stop asking.
Person says, "My mother is coming to see me," but the person's mother is dead.	Neither contradict the person nor play along. Try to respond to the general feeling of loss.
Person has a catastrophic reaction.	Do not ask questions. Slowly move the person to a private place. Stay calm and try to soothe the person. Under all circumstances, avoid arguing. Use simple distractions (e.g., "Let's go get a drink"). Touch the person and ask questions.

INAPPROPRIATE BEHAVIORS

As Alzheimer's disease progresses, more and more parts of the brain are destroyed. Eventually the person with Alzheimer's disease will become incontinent and unable to speak or walk. Ultimately the entire body will be affected and the person literally wastes away and dies at a weight of 70 or 80 pounds.

Part of the brain cell loss includes loss of impulse control. Infantile behaviors reappear. The person is no longer able to determine what behaviors are not socially acceptable (i.e., he or she may lose modesty, act out sexually, or become sloppy in appearance). The person loses sense of time and is unable to tolerate slight delays. He or she only experiences pain, pleasure, or discomfort, and may become insulting or curse when he or she perceives that needs have not been met.

The person with Alzheimer's disease is not at fault and cannot be expected to control his or her behavior. He or she may be craving more stimulation and attention and would respond well to a hug or pat or an opportunity to exercise moderately.

Coping Strategies for Caregivers

Being insulted or having to clean up smeared feces is always hard. There are times when a caregiver has to maintain a strong sense of humor and not take the remarks of the person with Alzheimer's disease personally.

People with Alzheimer's disease who are masturbating in public areas need to be taken to their own room (without blame or comment) unless they can be easily distracted from the activity. The caregiver must remember to stay calm when faced with this situation. Try not to draw attention to the person and give a false message of positive reinforcement (e.g., "Oh, look what Mr. Jones is doing!"). Masturbation is not an uncommon behavior and is acceptable if it is done in the individual's room. If the behavior is occurring frequently, be certain that the person does not have a urinary tract infection or skin excoriation in the perineal area.

Some of the coping strategies that are suggested for handling people with wandering behavior are also helpful for inappropriate behavior. Distraction is the key. Sharp retorts, scolding, and shaming are all nonproductive and frequently only serve to escalate the situation. The person with Alzheimer's disease will sense the caregiver's anger and disgust through body language. Laughter is a great antidote. Remember, the person is not to blame—the disease is.

Figures 4.2 and 4.3 are useful guides for two of the inappropriate behaviors that occur in people with Alzheimer's disease. They offer suggestions the caregiver can use to determine causes of incontinence and changes in sexual behavior. They also provide helpful interventions for these behaviors.

ANGER, AGGRESSION, AND CATASTROPHIC REACTIONS

Aggressive behavior usually occurs during the provision of personal or medical care. It is progressive. When people with Alzheimer's disease are not sure what is being said, their tension

Incontinence, which includes loss of bladder and/or bowel control and bedwetting, is a difficult problem if you're caring for an Alzheimer patient. Incontinence is common among Alzheimer patients—especially those in the latter stages of the disease.

Although you can manage incontinence by changing the patient's routine, clothing or environment, at some point you'll need to accept incontinence as a permanent condition of the disease.

If incontinence is a new behavior, your first and most important step is to identify the possible reasons for this loss of control. Ask yourself the following questions:

MEDICAL CONDITIONS

Could the reason be medical? For example, could the person have a urinary tract infection, constipation, or a prostate problem?

- Or is there an illness such as diabetes, stroke, or Parkinson's disease?
- Do movement difficulties make it hard for the patient to get to the bathroom in time? If the answer to any of these questions is "yes," you may want to consult with your physician.

STRESS

Is the incontinence caused by stress or movement? For example, does the person release urine with a sneeze, cough or laugh?

- Does fear of an embarrassing accident make the person want to continually visit the bathroom?
- Keep in mind weak pelvic muscles in a woman could cause uncontrollable loss of urine.

MEDICATION

Is the person on medication that might intensify the behavior?

- Is it possible that tranquilizers, sedatives, or diuretics contribute to incontinence? Keep in mind, for example, that some tranquilizers can relax the bladder muscles.
- Medications used to treat incontinence can cause such side effects as dry mouth and eye problems.

DEHYDRATION

Did you withhold fluids when the person started to lose bladder control? If so, the person might become dehydrated. Dehydration can, in turn, create a urinary tract infection which can lead to incontinence.

DIURETICS

Are you giving the person fluids that might produce a diuretic effect (increased urinating)? Beverages such as coffee, colas, and tea might contribute to incontinence.

(continued)

Figure 4.2.   Guidelines for incontinence. (From Alzheimer's Disease and Related Disorders Association, Inc. [1990]. *Incontinence.* Chicago: Author; reprinted by permission.)

Figure 4.2.   *(continued)*

ENVIRONMENT

Are there problems in the environment?

- Is it possible that the person can't find the bathroom? Does the person have too far to travel to reach the bathroom in time?
- Is the person afraid of falling? Are there obstacles in the path such as chairs or throw rugs? Is the path well lighted?

CLOTHING

Does the person have problems undressing in the bathroom? Are the zippers and buttons on clothing causing problems?

ACTION STEPS

Innovate

Be willing to experiment with new concepts and ideas. Keep in mind that every person is different. What works for one person may not work for another.

Understand

Remember that accidents are embarrassing. Be matter-of-fact and understanding and avoid blaming or scolding the individual.

- When the person is successful, use praise, encouragement and reassurance.

Communicate

Encourage the person to tell you when she thinks she needs to use the bathroom. The person may not be able to say, "I need to use the bathroom."

- Watch for visible cues that the person needs to use the bathroom. For example, the person may get restless, make unusual sounds or faces, or pace around the room.

Plan Ahead

Train yourself to respond to the person's routine and schedule. Identify when accidents occur and plan ahead.

- If an accident happens every two hours, you'll need to get the person to the bathroom before that time.
- You might also find it helpful to keep a notebook or log that notes when the person uses the bathroom.

Change and Adjust

Be patient and allow the person adequate time in the bathroom.

- In addition, rearrange the environment to make it easier for the person to use the bathroom. For example, leave on a nightlight in the bathroom and bedroom.
- Put a picture of a toilet on the bathroom door, or paint the bathroom door a color different than the wall.
- If accidents occur at night, consider a portable commode or urinal near the bed.

(continued)

Figure 4.2. *(continued)*

Simplify Clothing

Keep the person's dress simple and practical. Instead of choosing clothing with zippers and buttons, choose easy-to-remove and easy-to-clean styles such as sweat pants with elastic bands.

- Consider using such products as pads or protective bedding, adult diapers, or panty liners for female patients.

Follow-up

Make sure the person uses the bathroom. You may need to assist in removing clothes, wiping or flushing.

- You might also want to stimulate urination by giving the person a drink of water or running water in the sink.
- Keep sensitive skin areas clean with regular washing and application of a powder or ointment.

Control

To help control night incontinence, limit the person's intake of liquids after dinner and in the evening and cut down on drinks such as cola, coffee, tea, and grapefruit juice.

- Encourage the person to drink at least one-and-a-half quarts (six cups) of fluids daily. For variety, you might want to introduce decaffeinated herbal teas, decaffeinated coffee, Jell-O, or fruit juice.

Help the person with Alzheimer's retain a sense of dignity despite the problems with incontinence. Reassuring and non-judgmental statements will help lessen feelings of embarrassment.

---

and frustration escalate until they strike out. They seldom strike out in response to a simple "hello" from caregivers. In their confusion, people will respond with normal reactions to perceived danger. They strike out in self-defense. Some possible causes of anger, aggression, and catastrophic reactions in people with Alzheimer's disease include the following:

- Memory loss
- Inability to grasp what is going on or what is being said
- Inability to understand the concept of time
- Frustration at not being able to do what they were once capable of doing

Catastrophic reactions occur in situations that totally overwhelm people with Alzheimer's disease and cloud their abilities to understand and react normally. They overreact to simple incidents. Some examples of this type of reaction are extreme agitation, pacing, slamming doors or drawers, extreme stubbornness, intense crying, and striking out.

All human beings need to be touched, caressed and held. For Alzheimer patients and caregivers, this need is especially important. Alzheimer's disease affects people in varying ways. One person may have an increased interest in sex while another may have no interest. Changes in the sexuality of people with Alzheimer's disease include the following:

BOLD BEHAVIOR

The person may forget his or her marital status and begin to flirt or make inappropriate advances towards members of the opposite sex.

EXPOSURE

The person may forget how to dress or take her clothes off at inappropriate times and in unusual settings. For example, a woman or man may remove a blouse or shirt simply because it's too tight and she/he feels uncomfortable. The person doesn't realize or understand that clothes shouldn't be removed in public places.

FONDLING

The person may forget social rules or etiquette and fondle himself in public. Although it looks like the person is trying to harass or embarrass others, he really doesn't understand that his behavior is inappropriate.

PARANOIA

The person may become unreasonably jealous and suspicious. For example, the person may think that his wife has a boyfriend and accuse her of going to see him.

MISINTERPRETATIONS

The person may make sexual advances to a stranger who resembles a former spouse, lover or companion. In addition, the patient may forget that he or she is married and approach a person in a sexual manner.

PHYSICAL ILLNESS

Physical illness may cause the person to lose interest in sex or make sexual intercourse difficult or painful. Reactions to medications may also reduce sexual desire.

DEPRESSION

Depression can reduce interest in sex, both by the patient and their spouse or loved one. Some caregivers report that they experience changes in sexual feelings toward their loved ones after providing daily caretaking actions. By understanding these factors, and recognizing that they may affect you and the person with Alzheimer's, you will be able to respond better to the sexual needs of the person with Alzheimer's disease.

(continued)

Figure 4.3.   Guidelines for changes in sexuality. (From Alzheimer's Disease and Related Disorders Association, Inc. [1990]. *Changes in sexuality.* Chicago: Author; reprinted by permission.)

Figure 4.3.   *(continued)*

ACTION STEPS

Look for a Reason Behind the Behavior

Keep in mind that if the person exposes himself, he may simply need to go to the bathroom. If the person begins to take off his clothes, he may want to go to bed.

React to the Person with Patience and Gentleness

If the person is engaging in unusual sexual behavior, carefully remind her that the behavior is inappropriate. Then, lead the person to a private place or try to distract with another activity. But take care not to get angry with the person or laugh and giggle at the behavior. In most cases, anger and ridicule may cause negative reactions.

Respond Carefully to Threats and Accusations

If the person levels accusations or becomes extremely suspicious, don't waste time arguing. Instead, try to distract the person with another activity or reassure him with a hug or touch.

Adjust the Person's Clothing

Consider putting the person's trousers or dress on backward. Or provide the person with pull-on pants with no zipper.

Increase the Level of Appropriate Physical Contact

Give the person plenty of physical contact in the form of stroking, patting, hugging and rubbing. In many cases, the person is anxious and needs reassurance through touch and gentle, loving communication.

Adjust to Changes in Sexual Desire

As the disease progresses, a spouse may choose to sleep apart from the patient—especially if the person becomes overly demanding, jealous or irrational.

Seek Outside Help to Deal with Sexual Issues

If you consult an outside expert about sexual problems, make sure the professional understands the nature of the disease and will discuss sexual issues openly.

Coping Strategies for Caregivers

It is not always possible to prevent a catastrophic reaction. Each person with Alzheimer's disease is a unique individual and may react to a previously mild situation in a catastrophic way on a different day. Strategies for prevention of catastrophic reactions may include the following:

- Speak in simple, short sentences.
- Break large tasks into smaller ones. Smile and praise the person after he or she correctly performs each step.

- Give people time to respond after each direction; remember they think slowly.

- Repeat the directions exactly as given the first time, if they need to be repeated.

- Stop the discussion if the person becomes agitated or impatient. Come back in a few minutes and try again. The person will probably forget the previous encounter. However, if the caregivers have shown anger or impatience, the memory of those emotions may linger in the person's mind.

- Change or replace the caregiver.

- Continue on to another task, if completion of the task is not important.

- Stand close to people with Alzheimer's disease when giving personal care. Caregivers tend to stand far away in case the person hits or kicks. If the caregiver stands close and the person does strike out, the person's arm or leg will not be able to gain enough momentum to hurt the caregiver. Also, the caregiver will have time to stop the person or step back out of striking range.

If, despite your employment of good prevention strategies, a catastrophic reaction occurs, do the following:

- Remain calm. Speak quietly, but audibly. A reaction must be dealt with or it will get worse.

- Gently move the person to a quiet area—slowly and without pressure.

- Be soothing. Hold the person's hand. Pat him or her. Hug him or her gently.

- Feed the person. Food is used in many homes as a sign of caring and nurturing. Use cold foods in case the person throws or spills them. If possible, use cookie or cake items because sweets have a connotation of being a special treat.

- Try to determine what triggered the reaction when it is over so that the cause may be avoided in the future. People with Alzheimer's disease usually calm down as quickly as they flare up. Memory loss works for the caregiver's benefit as people quickly forget what just happened.

- Do not take the catastrophic reaction personally; it is simply a reaction to circumstances, not to a person.

Figure 4.4 identifies possible causes of frustration and combativeness with suggested interventions.

When an Alzheimer patient becomes combative, angry or agitated, it may be because of frustration. The individual may feel that he's being pushed to do something that simply can't be done.

Consider the following factors as possible sources of frustration:

DRESSING

The person who can't get his arm through a sweater may grow increasingly upset and start to thrash around.

BATHING

The person who's frightened by running water in the bathtub may push away a caregiver who's trying to give him a bath.

EATING

The person who doesn't like a certain type of food may refuse to eat it.

Keep in mind that combativeness takes many forms. Sometimes the person may simply try to push your hand away, while at other times the person may resist or strike you.

Deal with combativeness by trying to examine the underlying causes. Consider the following issues:

PHYSICAL CAUSES

Is the person tired because of inadequate rest or sleep? Are medications such as sedatives and tranquilizers creating side effects? Is the person unable to express the fact that he's in pain?

ENVIRONMENTAL CAUSES

Is the person overstimulated by loud noises, people or physical clutter? Is the environment unfamiliar? Does the person feel lost or abandoned by the caregiver?

POOR COMMUNICATION

Are you asking too many questions or making too many statements at once? Are your instructions simple and easy to understand? Is the person picking up on your own stress and irritability? Are you making the person more frustrated by being overly negative or critical?

ACTION STEPS

Be on the Lookout for Frustration
Look for early signs of frustration in such activities as bathing, dressing or eating, and respond in a calm and reassuring tone.

Don't Take Aggression and Combativeness Personally
Keep in mind that the person isn't necessarily angry at you. Instead, he may misunderstand the situation or be frustrated with his own disabilities.

(continued)

Figure 4.4.   Guidelines for combativeness. (From Alzheimer's Disease and Related Disorders Association, Inc. [1990]. *Combativeness.* Chicago: Author; reprinted by permission.)

Figure 4.4. *(continued)*

Avoid Teaching

Offer encouragement, but keep in mind the person's capabilities and don't expect more than he can do. Avoid elaborate explanations or arguments.

Use Distraction

Don't persist in making the person perform a particular task, especially if she has repeatedly been unsuccessful. If you see the person getting frustrated with buttoning a shirt, try to distract her with another activity such as putting on a pair of pants. After a time, you can return to the shirt. Or take the person to a quiet room, have a cup of tea, or go for a walk.

Communicate Directly with the Person

Avoid expressing anger or impatience in your voice or physical actions. Instead use positive, accepting expressions such as "please," "thank you," and "Don't worry, everything's going to be fine." In addition, use touch to reassure and comfort the person. For example, you might want to put your arm around the person or give him a kiss. In addition, follow these tips:

- Speak slowly and clearly.
- Use short, simple sentences.
- Approach the patient slowly and from the front.
- Use repetition and frequent reminders.

Decrease Your Level of Danger

Assess the level of danger—both for yourself and for the person. In other words, if the person becomes combative, ask this question: "How much trouble am I in—and what can I realistically do about it?" Often you can avoid harm by simply taking five steps back and standing away from the person for a short period of time. On the other hand, if the person is headed out of the house and onto a busy street, you need to be more aggressive.

Be Conservative in Using Restraint or Force

Unless the situation is serious, try to avoid physically holding or restraining the person. By fighting with the individual, you'll probably make him even more frustrated and anxious.

Experiment with Objects that Have a Soothing Effect

Some caregivers believe that stuffed animals have a soothing effect on the person, while others find that pets—from cats and dogs, to birds or goldfish—have a calming effect.

Learn from Previous Experiences

Try to avoid situations or experiences that make the person combative. For example, if the individual tires easily when she visits with family members, you might want to limit the length of these visits. Try to identify early signs of agitation: For example, outbursts are sometimes preceded by restlessness, frustration, fidgeting, or blushing.

Restructure Tasks and the Person's Environment

- Simplify tasks or plan more difficult tasks for the time of the day when the person is at his best.
- Give the person adequate time to respond to your directions or requests.
- Allow the person to make some choices, but limit the total number of choices. Having too many decisions to make about what to eat or wear might be confusing or overwhelming.
- Break down each task into small steps and allow the person to complete one step at a time.
- Keep the environment calm, quiet and clutter free.

UNIT 4: QUIZ

Please take a few minutes to complete the quiz for this unit. Answer each question as best you can. Keep in mind this is a learning tool to help you summarize and remember what has been discussed in this unit. For true-false questions, check the correct answer. For multiple choice questions, circle the correct answer(s).

Note: There may be more than one correct answer for some questions.

1. List three approaches to stop a person with Alzheimer's disease from wandering.

   a. _____

   b. _____

   c. _____

2. List three changes you can make in the person's environment that help prevent wandering.

   a. _____

   b. _____

   c. _____

3. People who wander usually are looking for someone or something they believe they have lost.

   ____ True   ____ False

4. Most aggressive behavior occurs while the caregiver is helping a person with activities of daily living.

   ____ True   ____ False

5. The best way to deal with a person who is exhibiting inappropriate sexual behavior is:

    a.   Tell the person to stop.

    b.   Give the person something to hold.

    c.   Take the person back to his or her room immediately.

    d.   Tie the person's hands loosely.

6. The most important thing to do when a person with Alzheimer's disease has a catastrophic reaction is to remain calm and _____.

7. People with Alzheimer's disease usually hit caregivers because _____.

8. Physical restraints do not help develop a person's sense of cooperation because they do not help develop a sense of trust between the person with Alzheimer's disease and the caregiver.

    ____ True   ____ False

9. All behavior has significance.

    ____ True   ____ False

UNIT 4: INSTRUCTOR HELP

1. Audiovisuals

   a. Two videotapes from the University of Washington are available: "Managing Aggressive Behaviors: Anger, Irritation and Catastrophic Reactions" (20 minutes) and "Managing Difficult Behaviors: Wandering and Inappropriate Sexual Behaviors" (19 minutes).

   b. One transparency from Table 4.1 is provided for this session. Place a piece of paper on top of the Suggested Solutions column and ask the trainees to offer suggestions to each of the situations presented in the Situation column. If they are unable to offer a solution or after some discussion, uncover the Suggested Solutions column and discuss these. Make note of useful suggestions offered by the class for use at another session.

2. Discussion/questions

   a. Difficult behaviors are hot topics for caregivers and discussion probably will generate itself. You may wish to have the trainees discuss some solutions that have worked for them when they dealt with these behaviors.

   b. It is important to deal with the caregiver's feeling about these difficult behaviors (e.g., anger, frustration, embarrassment).

   c. Caregivers sometimes try to deal with behaviors such as wandering by restraining the individual with Alzheimer's disease. Although the author does not believe that this is the appropriate response to wandering and many alternative methods are suggested, occasionally a staff member can benefit from the actual experience of being restrained for even a brief period of time. If you select this experience for your trainees, it is very important for participants to share their feelings afterward. Otherwise, the point is lost.

   d. Role-play situations are useful. This helps trainees develop skills in "what to say" and "how to say it."

Unit 5

Medications for Depression and Behavior Amelioration

Learning Objectives

1. To understand how aging affects the body's ability to tolerate medications

2. To understand the appropriate role of medications in treating depression and managing behavior in people with Alzheimer's disease

3. To cite the benefits of medications in people with Alzheimer's disease

4. To be able to recognize common side effects of medications used to treat depression and behavior

There are many normal physiological changes of aging that alter the older person's ability to tolerate, utilize, and eliminate drugs. This is true of all medications, not just ones prescribed for depression and behavior change. Therefore, it is important for caregivers to be aware of the physiological changes that affect the way the body handles medications.

PHARMACOKINETICS AND AGING

Pharmacokinetics is the name of the processes by which the body absorbs, distributes, metabolizes, and eliminates medications. Pharmacokinetics is affected by gastrointestinal changes, changes in body composition, liver function, and renal function.

Gastrointestinal Changes

The ability to absorb medications into the body water and the body fat from the upper gastrointestinal tract is unchanged in the older adult. Absorption is affected by changes in gastrointestinal motility. Some medications slow gastrointestinal movement, allowing more time for absorption to occur and therefore increasing their effects. Medications taken for depression and psychosis (tricyclic antidepressants and phenothiazines), allergies and congestion (antihistamines), and intestinal or bladder spasms (anticholinergics) slow gastrointestinal motility. Laxatives increase gastrointestinal motility and may prevent adequate absorption of other medications, thus reducing their effects.

Older people frequently exhibit a decreased production of hydrochloric acid in the stomach (hypochlorhydria). Some medications, such as phenobarbital, require the presence of hydrochloric acid in order to begin breaking down prior to being metabolized. If there is inadequate hydrochloric acid present, the benefit from some medications may be decreased.

Other age-related changes that might alter medication absorption include decreased blood flow to the gastrointestinal tract, especially the small intestine. In most cases, the age-related changes in the gastrointestinal tract do not significantly affect medication absorption.

Changes in Body Composition

There are several age-related changes in body composition that can significantly alter the distribution of medications in the body. The proportion of body fat increases, and total body water, plasma volume, and extracellular fluid decrease. The reduction in lean body mass affects distribution of medications by decreasing the area (volume) within which distribution can occur, thereby producing high peak levels. The reduction in total body water may cause water-soluble medications such as lithium and salicylates to reach dangerous (toxic) levels in the bloodstream.

Increased body fat raises one's ability to store fat-soluble compounds such as benzodiazepines and phenothiazines and increases the risk of toxicity as doses accumulate. This means that over time, more medication is accumulated than is eliminated from the body. Blood levels rise and undesirable (toxic) side effects may occur. The following medications are some of the most likely to accumulate and cause toxicity: Valium, Dalmane, Restoril, and Halcion.

Concentration of an important protein in the blood, serum albumin, decreases slightly with age. Many older people are nutritionally protein deficient because they cannot chew meat, cannot afford foods with protein, or have decreased appetites. In these people, medications that must attach to a protein to be transported to the sites in the body where they can be effective will not have sufficient protein attachments. This situation causes increased amounts of the medication to be free in the circulation and is likely to cause toxic side effects. Propanolol (Inderal), phenytoin (Dilantin), and most antibiotics are highly protein-bound.

Other factors to consider when giving medication to older adults are reduced cardiac output and the increase in peripheral vascular resistance. Blood flow to the liver and kidney decreases and more of the cardiac output is distributed to the skeletal muscle and cerebral and coronary areas.

Changes in Liver Function

Liver metabolism is also affected by the decrease in blood flow and the decrease in liver mass. Medications that are given orally are particularly affected by these liver changes. An age-related reduction in liver microsomal enzymatic activity and inducibility has been found that may lead to reduced medication metabolism and increased medication accumulation and toxicity.

Medications that have been demonstrated to have a decreased metabolic effect on the liver in older adults include diazepam and theophylline. The implication is that older people require smaller doses of these medications to prevent toxicity.

Changes in Renal Function

There is approximately a 1% loss per year in renal (kidney) function after about age 40. As a result, medications that are excreted primarily by certain structures in the kidney are removed more slowly and less completely. Various disease states, such as congestive heart failure and dehydration, further reduce renal blood flow and the rate at which medications are excreted.

Creatinine is a substance produced by the normal breakdown of body protein (muscle mass). It can be found in the blood (serum) and the urine and is a measure of renal function. In older adults, the serum level of creatinine may be normal even in the presence of abnormal kidney function. It is much more accurate to measure the amount of creatinine present in a 24-hour collection of urine. This measurement is called *creati-*

nine clearance. If the kidneys are not functioning well, the creatinine clearance will be low. This affects the elimination time of medications and may result in increased blood levels of medications (and possible toxicity) and require longer periods for medications to be completely eliminated.

In general, dosage guidelines for medications ordered for older people cut the starting dose in half for people over 65 years of age and cut them by three fifths for people 85 years and older. The motto is "Start low and go slow."

SIGNS AND SYMPTOMS OF REACTIONS TO MEDICATION AND INTERACTIONS

Unwanted side effects of medications are seven times more common in older adults than in younger adults. The likelihood of two or more medications acting together to cause unwanted side effects (interactions) also increases in the older person. There are several reasons for this besides the fact that pharmacokinetics change. Older people tend to have more chronic illnesses that may be treated with one or more medications. Many pharmacologists believe that if a person is taking more than three medications, including vitamins and antacids, it is hard to determine if any medication is truly treating a disease process or a drug interaction. For example, if an older person is taking three or four medications for disease symptoms, it is very likely a drug interaction will occur, causing one or more additional symptoms. The response by the physician to these new symptoms may be to prescribe another medication. This new medication may, in turn, cause another drug interaction, thus causing additional symptoms. Soon it becomes difficult to determine which, if any, medication is treating a disease symptom and which is treating a drug interaction.

Older people are not often helped to understand how to take a medication properly and the doctor does not always ask if the person can afford the prescription. Consequently, there is much room for error. Many medications are very expensive. As a result, older people may stop taking a medication as soon as they feel better. They may decide to try it again several months or years later when similar symptoms reappear. By then, the medication is outdated or is not correct for the problem. More than 25% of emergency room admissions for people over age 65 are for drug reactions or drug interactions. The older person who is at highest risk for these adverse effects would have one or more of the following characteristics:

- Small stature (5 feet, 2 inches or shorter)
- A positive history of allergic illness
- A documented history of previous reactions to medications
- Multiple chronic illnesses
- Renal or hepatic (liver) impairment
- Involvement of more than one physician and pharmacist in care
- Atypical mental status
- Solitary living
- Financial difficulty
- A visual or hearing impairment

Caregivers should closely observe people who are taking medications and be aware of any signs of a reaction. Signs to watch for include the following:

- Confusion and/or agitation
- Orthostatic hypotension (i.e., feeling faint when standing up due to drop in blood pressure)
- Hypothermia
- Pseudo-Parkinsonism/tardive dyskinesia (tongue movements, lip smacking, teeth grinding, finger movements that imitate "pill rolling")
- Constipation
- Lethargy
- Anorexia (i.e., decreased appetite)
- Dry mouth
- Dizziness
- Urinary retention
- Weight gain

PHARMACOLOGICAL INTERVENTIONS FOR BEHAVIOR AND MOOD PROBLEMS

Nonpharmacological treatments should be given a fair trial before utilizing medications when a person with Alzheimer's disease experiences behavior problems (see Unit 4). Nonpharmacological interventions, such as distracting, providing a structured environment, and interacting person to person more frequently, usually take longer to show results, but the extra time is well worth it. Change may require 4 or more weeks to be noticeable. People with moderate to severe Alzheimer's disease will require a longer time period to become comfortable in new surroundings. Sometimes 4–6 weeks is necessary for the adjustment. The more severe the Alzheimer's disease, the longer the adjustment period. Sometimes the undesired behavior is self-limited and will disappear within a couple of weeks. As people with dementia pass through the worsening stages, behaviors change and, again, often go away within a short time. There is the reality, however, that people who are dangerous to themselves and/or others must be treated sooner with chemical interventions.

Sometimes tranquilizers and antidepressants are used unethically and improperly as chemical restraints. They are used in doses that keep people sedated, confused, and less active. This is a totally unacceptable practice! At various times, it is tempting to quiet a person with Alzheimer's disease who may be loud or aggressive. As previously stated, behavioral interventions should be tried before medications are used, however (see Unit 4).

Behaviors that are commonly seen during the early stages of Alzheimer's disease and particularly after moving to a new location are those that accompany depression. People who are depressed do not smile very often, usually have poor appetites, are often confused, and express thoughts of worthlessness or wanting to die. They may be lethargic—not wanting to participate in any activities or do things for themselves—or they may become agitated and rather hyperactive. These signs must be present for more than 2 weeks before the condition can be named clinical depression.

There are other processes besides Alzheimer's disease that cause depression. These include hypothyroidism and diabetes, and drug reactions and interactions. When determining the cause of the person's changed behaviors, it is important to rule out physical causes of depression. It also is important to diagnose the mood problem accurately so that the most appropriate medication is selected. Occasionally, psychiatric intervention is necessary.

Tranquilizers such as Haldol and Mellaril must be started in very small doses and raised in small increments no more frequently than every 5–7 days. This length of time is necessary to reach a steady pharmacological state. Doses should be increased only until there is a satisfactory change in behavior. Older people frequently do not need to be within the therapeutic plasma level in order to derive excellent benefits from a medication. If the dosage is increased until the person enters the therapeutic range, drug toxicity is often the result.

Some common side effects of major tranquilizers (e.g., haloperidol, thorazine) include the following:

- Orthostatic hypotension
- Urinary retention
- Constipation
- Dry mouth
- Elevated intraocular pressure (i.e., glaucoma)
- Blurred vision
- Akathisia (i.e., muscle restlessness and inability to sit upright)
- Tardive dyskinesia
- Parkinsonism (i.e., muscular rigidity, tremors)
- Paradoxical reactions (i.e., increased agitation, restlessness, confusion, and disorientation)

Drug Benefits

If a medication for a mood disorder is appropriately selected, the person will have an enhanced sense of well-being, decreased anxiety and restlessness, and may sleep better. The incidence of hallucinations and paranoia should decrease. If the person responds paradoxically (i.e., the opposite of what you expect) or the wrong drug is selected, mood and behavior problems may increase. The solution to this is to stop the drug. The person's physician must be consulted before stopping medications for mood disorders. Most of these medications should be stopped gradually rather than abruptly in order to avoid undesirable side effects.

Antidepressant Medications

Antidepressant medications can be helpful in the early stages of Alzheimer's disease or other types of dementia. During the early periods, the person has sufficient cognitive function to understand that he or she has an incurable, progressive, debilitating disease. Sadness is a normal response to such an impending loss. If the depression is severe enough to cause harm to the person (e.g., anorexia, refusal to drink or move), the temporary use of an antidepressant is helpful. Antidepressants can help to rule out depression as an underlying cause of the dementia symptoms.

Like some tranquilizers, antidepressants need to be prescribed initially in small doses and slowly increased to a therapeutic dosage for the individual. Recently, a new class of antidepressant has become available, called the selective serotonin reuptake inhibitors (SSRIs). This class was tested on older people during early clinical trials. There were few side effects and very little of the dry mouth, tardive dyskinesia, and other anticholinergic properties that accompany the tricyclic antidepressants. Some antidepressants most commonly prescribed include the following:

- Desyrel (trazodone): tricyclic
- Sinequan (doxepin): tricyclic
- Norpramin (desipramine): tricyclic
- Prozac (fluoxetine): SSRI
- Zoloft (sertraline): SSRI
- Paxil (paroxetine): SSRI

Some major side effects of antidepressants include the following:

- Sedation
- Orthostatic hypotension
- Constipation
- Dry mouth
- Blurred vision
- Urinary retention
- Anorexia

The following is a list for proper use and precautions with antidepressants:

- Medication should be taken with food to decrease the possibility of gastric upset.
- Medication should be taken at bedtime to enhance sedative effects. If nightmares or postural hypotension occurs, a half dose should be taken at bedtime and the remainder during the day.
- Small doses (two fifths to half of the usual adult dose) are recommended in initial therapy with small increments until

the optimum dose is achieved. Liquid formulations may be used to provide for smaller doses.

- Optimum effects of the medication may not occur for 4–6 weeks.

- Medication should not be discontinued without discussing the change with a physician.

- The physician or dentist should be alerted about the person's medication prior to surgeries.

- The person should avoid drinking alcohol.

- Medication in an oral liquid form should not be taken with grape juice or carbonated beverages because this may reduce the effectiveness.

- To prevent sudden dizziness, the person should be advised to rise slowly from lying to sitting to standing.

- Drug interactions can occur with most other medications, especially blood pressure medications and seizure medications. Be sure to ask the health care provider or the pharmacist about possible interactions with other medicines the person may be taking.

ADMINISTERING MEDICATIONS

Only caregivers or the staff who have been authorized and taught proper doses and procedures may administer medicine to people with Alzheimer's disease, and only a health care provider can prescribe medications. At times, administering medication can be a very frustrating and confrontational experience. People with Alzheimer's disease will sometimes take medications from certain nurses and not from others.

One of the keys to success is communication technique. Try to find and utilize the person's remaining capacities to help build trust. Searching for the meaning behind the behavior may help you to understand, for example, that a belligerent person with Alzheimer's disease is objecting only to taking the medication with his or her meal instead of before the meal. Emotions are used to express this desire because he or she cannot find the words to communicate in any other way.

When administering medications, always observe the person taking it. Never leave the dose with the person and walk away. Offer plenty of plain water or juice with the medication (i.e., 6–8 ounces) to ensure that the medication does not remain in the esophagus where it may cause harm. Be sure to consult with a pharmacist before crushing pills or opening capsules. Learn the idiosyncrasies of the person's medication-taking behavior and be as flexible as you can about the timing. If the person refuses the medication, do not force the issue but try again later. This will avoid confrontation and a "no-win" situation.

Sometimes medications can be mixed with food (e.g., applesauce, pudding, Jell-O, jelly) to make them more palatable. However, deceiving the person with Alzheimer's disease by saying that the medication is dessert or tastes good or by otherwise camouflaging the medication may ultimately backfire and make the person distrust you. He or she may accuse you of poisoning him or her or refuse to eat.

Finally, and possibly most importantly, ask the health care provider whether or not the person really needs the medication. Would he or she be just as well off without it? It is always good practice to keep the number of medications given to a minimum. Be sure to report and record the person's responses to medications, especially if you suspect an adverse response.

UNIT 5: QUIZ

Please take a few minutes to complete the quiz for this unit. Answer each question as best you can. Keep in mind this is a learning tool to help you summarize and remember what has been discussed in this unit. For true-false questions, check the correct answer. For multiple choice questions, circle the correct answer(s).

Note: There may be more than one correct answer for some questions.

1. List three side effects of tricyclic antidepressants.

   a. _____

   b. _____

   c. _____

2. For older people, the starting dose of an antidepressant or tranquilizer should be about two fifths to half that of the recommended adult starting dose.

   ____ True   ____ False

3. Anorexia, lethargy, and increased confusion are common symptoms of drug interaction or toxicity.

   ____ True   ____ False

4. If you are administering medications and a person who had a diagnosis of Alzheimer's disease said "Those are not my pills," what would you do?

   a. Argue that they were indeed his or her pills and administer them.

   b. Recheck the medication sheet for changes.

   c. Agree with the person, but try later to administer the same pills, believing that he or she would forget what he or she had said.

   d. None of the above.

5. Overdose or medication interactions can cause symptoms
    of dementia in otherwise normal people.

    ____ True   ____ False

6. Tardive dyskinesia is best defined as:

    a. Increased confusion in the person.

    b. A seizure disorder caused by medications.

    c. Involuntary muscle movements caused by long-term
        use of certain medications.

    d. Inability to sit upright unless supported.

7. Haldol is a dangerous medication and should seldom be
    used to treat behaviors in people with dementia.

    ____ True   ____ False

8. Sleep disturbances in the person with dementia are best
    treated with:

    a. Behavioral intervention.

    b. Chloral hydrate.

    c. Halcion.

    d. A glass of wine.

UNIT 5: INSTRUCTOR HELP

This session is probably best taught by a licensed nurse or pharmacist. It applies primarily to licensed staff (and medication technicians, if you have them), but all facility personnel could benefit from knowing about some of the side effects of medications. If they are informed, they can be helpful in the monitoring process. If you want to teach the side effects portion of this chapter to unlicensed staff, you may wish to add it to another session that is short. The side effects discussion probably will not take more than 15 minutes.

1. Audiovisuals

There are no supplemental materials designed for this session. It could be useful to prepare a one- or two-page handout on the drug interactions and side effects of the medications most commonly used with people with Alzheimer's disease in your facility.

2. Discussion/questions

Much of this unit does not lend itself to discussion. Remain open to questions during the presentation. Discussion might be useful regarding the answers to the quiz questions or when talking about helpful hints for getting people with difficult behaviors to take medications.

Unit 6

Supporting the Caregivers— Families and Staff

Learning Objectives

1. To recognize signs of stress that may be experienced by the staff or primary caregiver
2. To list some techniques that may be used by either the staff or a family member to cope with their own negative feelings
3. To state two ways the staff can help family caregivers
4. To know what information staff should seek from family

Much has been written about caregivers of people with Alzheimer's disease, but very little has been done to address the stress and burnout experienced by a staff member or family member working with people with Alzheimer's disease. It is not unreasonable to assume that the staff experience many of the same feelings as family members.

CARING FOR STAFF

Caring for a person with dementia is physically and emotionally exhausting work. Sometimes a staff member can be his or her "own worst enemy." It is easy to become very emotionally attached to people with Alzheimer's disease, especially when a staff member works with them on a day-to-day basis. Sometimes staff members think that no one else can care as well as they can. This belief can prevent staff members from recognizing their own stress levels and from being willing to take an easier assignment until they are emotionally ready.

Recognizing Stress

If the frustration experienced by the staff who care for people with Alzheimer's disease is not handled, the staff member may experience burnout. Burnout is a result of physical and emotional exhaustion. The caregiver withdraws from all emotional reaction (i.e., just does the job) and lacks any spontaneity or enthusiasm. Signs of stress are experienced by both staff and family members. The following is a list of symptoms of stress and burnout:

Anger is felt if the staff member believes the person is behaving in a particular way on purpose. The staff member may also feel anger if the person never expresses appreciation for best efforts, or if the staff member dislikes a particular task (e.g., cleaning up after incontinence).

Helplessness is felt if the staff member does not understand the person's behavior or reaction, or if the staff member does not know how to help the person.

Embarrassment is felt in response to socially unacceptable behavior acted out by the person (e.g., masturbation, incontinence).

Guilt is experienced if the person never improves and must be moved to a different level of care.

Grief occurs when a person must be moved to a different level of care.

Depression is experienced when a person's health deteriorates or he or she dies. It can also occur in relation to the overall care requirements of people with Alzheimer's disease.

Isolation results from thinking that other care providers do not experience the same negative feelings, causing the caregiver to feel alone or isolated. The staff person may feel that there is nowhere to go for help in dealing with a person with Alzheimer's disease.

Concern is felt from never knowing "if I did enough," or realizing that no emotional reaction is occurring from the person.

Physical reactions to stress may be manifested by an increase in fatigue, vague physical complaints such as headaches, gastrointestinal disturbances, and illness that may result in increased sick time.

Helping the Staff Cope

There are ways a care facility can help caregivers alleviate some feelings of frustration and burnout. Suggestions offered include the following:

- Recognize negative feelings. It is not uncommon for caregivers to feel frustrated or angry, or to feel overwhelmed by caring for people with Alzheimer's disease. If these feelings are not recognized, they can negatively influence the way the caregiver cares for the person. If the feelings are recognized, the caregiver will be able to respond more rationally to the person with Alzheimer's disease and can begin to do something to alleviate the feelings.

- Encourage open, honest communications among caregivers. Provide opportunities for staff to share with peers good and bad experiences and their reactions to them. Any staff member (e.g., dietary, housekeeping) who comes in contact with people with Alzheimer's disease or families should be invited to participate in these sharing groups.

- Provide regular inservice training. The staff need a variety of management techniques from which to choose. Inservices work most effectively if the staff have an opportunity to try out the learned techniques, and then return another time and discuss how the techniques did or did not work.

- Establish support groups. Focus on feelings and techniques to manage or prevent the negative feelings. Focus on ethical issues. There are times when a staff member's personal ethics may create stress and conflict among other caregivers. Focus on care management issues and stress reduction techniques. The difference in these support groups is that the group is made up of peers rather than all staff.

- Ensure respite for staff. Rotate staff to units where people are in less severe stages of Alzheimer's disease, increase contact with families to enhance staff person's sense of accomplishment, change responsibilities sometimes, and give staff an opportunity to lead an activity—this offers them more social interaction.

- Offer a trial period to new employees. Be sure new employees can cope successfully and offer reassurance that they can transfer if they cannot cope.

Table 6.1 lists symptoms of burnout; Table 6.2 offers a quick reference for avoiding burnout.

Table 6.1.   Symptoms of burnout experienced by caregivers

• Absenteeism	• Impatience
• Avoidance	• Irritability
• Chronic fatigue	• Lack of enthusiasm
• Depression	• Physical complaints

CARING FOR FAMILIES

The majority of people with Alzheimer's disease are cared for at home by family members. These family members do not always know what type of community assistance is available. They also may not have other relatives or friends nearby to assist with care. Some caregivers are too embarrassed by the behaviors of the person with Alzheimer's disease and do not want anyone else to see these behaviors. Often the person with Alzheimer's disease has disrupted sleep patterns and the caregiver is only able to sleep for short periods of time. Every task (e.g., grocery shopping, housecleaning, cooking) is difficult because there are so many interruptions. Sometimes the doctor prescribes sleeping medicine for the person with Alzheimer's disease so the caregiver can get some sleep. However, the person may react severely to the medicine and become lethargic

Table 6.2.   Suggestions for caregivers for avoiding burnout

1. Know what makes you angry or impatient. List 10 things, beginning with those that are most upsetting.
2. Use mental imagery or visualization to see yourself successfully handling a stressful situation. Imagine how someone you most admire might handle the situation. What techniques did the person use?
3. Use self-talk, which is a powerful tool. Say to yourself, "I will not let this upset me."
4. Evaluate the situation objectively. Is the person behaving reasonably, given the reality of the situation?
5. Be flexible. "Go with the flow."
6. Make a list of prioritizing tasks, but do not agonize over unexpected crises.
7. Develop effective management techniques based on sound knowledge of Alzheimer's disease.
8. Balance expectations of the job with expectations of home, family, and friends. Do not try to be all things to all people. Let others help, especially at home.
9. Take care of yourself physically, mentally, and spiritually. Eat well. Plan time for exercise, relaxation, meditation, and other activities that interest you.
10. Praise your own special skills and understand clearly what your tasks entail.

and not eat or drink for several days. Now the caregiver is worried that the person has become ill.

These are very typical scenarios in families, especially when a person is caring for a spouse with Alzheimer's disease, the children are grown and living far away, and friends are too old to help with care. The entire burden is on the spouse who is healthy.

A healthy spouse or caregiver experiences the same emotions the staff in a care facility do: anger, helplessness, embarrassment, guilt, grief, depression, isolation, concern, and constant fatigue.

Finally, the person with Alzheimer's disease reaches a stage when placement in a care facility is considered seriously by the healthy spouse. Increased need for physical or medical care, incontinence, wandering, assaultive behavior, and exhaustion felt by the caregiver may precipitate placement. Home care lasts 24 hours every day while care in a facility is broken into 8-hour shifts.

Care at home can be prolonged if the caregiver has some outside support, either from friends and family or an agency. Respite care to allow the caregiver to sleep, go outside the home on errands, or attend a support group for caregivers of people with Alzheimer's disease can make an immeasurable difference in the physical and emotional well-being of the caregiver.

Support groups sponsored by the Alzheimer's Disease and Related Disorders Association are especially helpful. The caregiver learns about the disease from an accurate source. Caregivers share ideas and tips and emotional support and advice is given regarding legal matters and placement in a care facility. The caregiver is referred to other agencies as needed for home care and financial assistance. Sometimes day care is provided for the ill spouse during the support group meeting.

Family response to placing a person with Alzheimer's disease in a nursing home can be intense. There are many concerns that need to be addressed. The healthy spouse has been the main provider of care for a long time and worries that the nursing home staff will not know how to care for his or her spouse. The healthy spouse thinks about all the other people the staff have to care for and wonders if there will be time to check on his or her spouse. Feelings of relief are often mixed with feelings of guilt about leaving a spouse in the care of strangers. Sometimes the spouse's behavior is embarrassing and the healthy spouse wonders if the staff will understand and accept these strange behaviors.

Working with Family Members

It is critical that staff and family members learn to work together in the care of a person with Alzheimer's disease. Families have a wealth of information regarding a person's idiosyncrasies and past life patterns. Families who have cared for the person with Alzheimer's disease for months or years can tell staff what techniques work best to prevent catastrophic reactions and get the person to eat. The staff are helpful because they can provide a wealth of information on management techniques and explaining the changes that are occurring in the person.

The person with Alzheimer's disease will benefit when the staff and family work together. Suggestions to help staff and family work together include the following:

• Open lines of communication. Encourage the family to ask questions and allow family members to express feelings about placement. Be supportive. Express interest in the person's past history. Take time to listen.

• Make the family's visit pleasant. Explain the routines of the facility. If there are activities in the daily care routine in which family members can participate, encourage them to do so. Sometimes a family is reluctant to visit. Family members may wish to remember the person "as she was." Help them to see the value of the visit, yet remember that visits may be very difficult for them.

• Give information to the family caregiver. Explain changes that are occurring as a result of the disease process. Help the family see that behavior problems are a result of the illness.

• Remind family of the person's capabilities. Explain that due to communication problems, he or she may understand more than he or she is able to express.

• Request information from the family caregiver. Collect information concerning past history and behavior. Inquire about the person's employment, children, and hobbies. This can help the staff person understand the person's behaviors later. Also, find out what the family has tried regarding behavior management, especially what has been effective. This will help the person and staff.

Table 6.3 is a list of the types of information the caregiving staff and the family can share—all for the benefit of the person with Alzheimer's disease.

Table 6.3.   Caregiving staff and families—what each can tell the other

What caregiving staff can tell families	What families can tell staff
• Program routines	• Cultural background
• Visits and participation in programs are welcomed	• Spiritual beliefs
• Interested in the patient	• Educational background
• Specific activities families might participate in with the person	• Previous occupations
• Information about the disease process	• Hobbies
• Changes that are occurring	• Area where the person spent most of his or her life
• Therapeutic changes	• Family/marriage
• Short-term goals for the person	• Children: names, ages, jobs, location
• Plans for the person	• Grandchildren
• Person's adjustment to the program	• Siblings: names, locations
• Signs of positive change	• Special friends
• Value of caregiver's visits	• Special qualities, abilities (past/present)
• Strengths in the person	• Food likes and dislikes
• Friendships, relationships that have been established	• Person's attitude about losses, changes
	• Person's expectations of the placement
	• Past effective techniques for managing disruptive behavior

UNIT 6: QUIZ

Please take a few minutes to complete the quiz for this unit. Answer each question as best you can. Keep in mind this is a learning tool to help you summarize and remember what has been discussed in this unit. For true-false questions, check the correct answer. For multiple choice questions, circle the correct answer(s).

Note: There may be more than one correct answer for some questions.

1. The staff and family members experience many of the same feelings and frustrations.

    _____ True   _____ False

2. List three signs of stress that may be experienced by either the staff or the family member.

    a. _____

    b. _____

    c. _____

3. Which of the following statements concerning interaction between the staff and family members is incorrect?

    a. The family may provide information as to effective ways to handle the person's behavior.

    b. It is helpful for the staff member to express his or her dislike of the person to the family.

    c. The staff may help the family member to make future plans.

    d. The family may provide a staff member with information about the person's past likes and dislikes.

4. Which of the following statements concerning the handling of a staff member's feelings is incorrect?

    a. Anger should not be expressed and should be internalized.

    b. Meetings should be scheduled to discuss the people with Alzheimer's disease and care issues.

    c. Staff should recognize that they can and do experience negative feelings about certain people.

    d. Support groups should be conducted to facilitate open communication.

5. At the time of placement in a care facility, the primary caregiver may be experiencing all of the following emotions: relief, frustration, sadness, and anger.

    ____ True   ____ False

6. Physical reactions such as fatigue, headaches, gastrointestinal disturbance, and constipation may be an indication of job stress for staff members.

    ____ True   ____ False

7. List three ways the staff can help primary (family) caregivers adjust to placing a family member with Alzheimer's disease in a nursing home.

    a. _____

    b. _____

    c. _____

8. List two situations when it is beneficial for the staff person to request information from the primary caregiver.

    a. _____

    b. _____

UNIT 6: INSTRUCTOR HELP

1. Audiovisuals
   a. Two transparencies are provided for this session. Use Symptoms of Burnout to ask the trainees if they have ever experienced these symptoms. Use the second transparency excerpted from Table 6.2 to discuss suggestions for avoiding burnout. This can be used to begin the discussion in 2b below.
   b. A videotape from the University of Washington titled "Caregiver Issues" (30 minutes) is available. Be sure you preview the videotape to identify the parts you want to emphasize.

2. Discussion/questions
   a. In general, people usually are willing to discuss feelings of burnout. You should be able to generate a good discussion about staff burnout and working with families.
   b. Staff burnout is an important topic and there probably will be little coaxing needed for the trainees to tell you (and each other) what strategies could be used to help them avoid burnout.

Unit 7

Special Care Units

Approximately 50% of nursing home admissions in the United States are due to progressive dementias, with Alzheimer's disease representing the largest proportion of those dementias. This population of institutionalized older people will increase in number as the total U.S. population ages.

The nursing home industry is making great efforts to provide quality care for these individuals. The newest trend to evolve is the special care unit. This unit exists independently or can be incorporated into an already established nursing home.

BENEFITS OF SPECIAL CARE UNITS

Special care units have some distinct advantages over traditional nursing care facilities. For example, in a nursing home people with good cognitive function are mixed with people with dementia; however, these same people would be separated in a special care unit according to their level of dementia. Some of the advantages of a special care unit include the following:

- Distractions and confusing stimuli are minimized. Noises, such as overhead paging and background music, are eliminated in special care units. Furnishings in the living areas are colorful, and are either plain or have a simple pattern so they are not confusing to a person with dementia.

- Professional staff are recruited and trained specifically to care for people with Alzheimer's disease and other dementias. Staff in special care units usually receive more hours of training and training that is more specialized in caring for people with dementia.

- Activities are more individualized. Special care units have a greater number of staff per resident. With more activities staff per person, each person receives more attention and a greater amount of one-to-one time.

- Chemical and physical restraints are used only minimally. Several factors contribute to a greater capability to utilize behavioral interventions. The environment is designed to be accommodating to people with dementia, such as the freedom to wander without becoming lost or injuring themselves. More staff per person allow caregivers to devote more attention to the individuals' needs. Staff have received, and continue to receive, specific training in how to manage difficult behaviors.

• Nutritional status is improved. The kinds of foods served and the way in which they are served is more accommodating for people with dementia. For example, finger foods are served, people are allowed to wander while they eat, foods are available at all times (not just at mealtimes), and foods high in calories are served to replace the calories used in the greater degree of activity for people who wander.

• Agitation and wandering are reduced. People are allowed to move about freely and unattended, which causes the muscles to tire and thus produces a calming effect. Also, people with similar degrees of dementia can relate to one another and seem to enjoy interacting even though the conversations may make no sense to the caregiver. This interaction is also calming to the individuals.

• Caregivers work more directly with the families. The smaller number of caregivers per person allows the caregivers to become more involved with the individuals and their families. Additionally, the caregivers have been taught the importance of family involvement and are, therefore, inclined to encourage family involvement.

Special care units do have some drawbacks. Recruiting staff is problematic because caring for people with dementia is frustrating—the disease does not improve and often makes no sense. It takes a special person to care for people with dementia, meaning rather unique individuals have to be recruited. Another drawback is the cost. These units are often more costly than traditional nursing homes, which is not surprising because the staff to resident ratio is higher. Generally, however, special care units provide a better quality of care for people with dementia than traditional nursing homes.

BASIC PROVISIONS OF SPECIAL CARE UNITS

There can be vast differences among special care units. Some are considered locked units within existing facilities that are designed to manage safely the person with dementia who wanders. Other units are physically separate from other facilities. Provisions of special care units for a comfortable environment for both the caregiver and the person with Alzheimer's disease include the following:

- A cheerful, home-like atmosphere with the person's personal mementos is created. It is important to have a comfortable, homey atmosphere that includes items such as furnishings and pictures from the person's own home and family.

- Cheerful living areas that are not distracting are designed. Care should be taken in selecting wallpaper, floor covering, and furniture coverings so that they are attractive, but not confusing. For example, wallpaper with flowers and vines could be very confusing to a person with dementia. Mirrored walls would also be very confusing.

- Living areas are safe and well lit. The residents need to be able to walk about freely without risk of injuring themselves.

- Pleasant odors are evident. It is important the environment be pleasant in appearance and scent. Unpleasant odors are not only distasteful to both the caregiver and the person with Alzheimer's disease, but can be distracting and confusing to the person with dementia.

- Noise and confusion levels are reduced. Busy activity areas, such as bathing rooms and laundry areas, are located away from individuals' rooms. Living areas are peaceful, with minimal noise and confusion generated by caregivers and visitors.

- Music is provided, but little or no overhead paging is heard. Music may be provided, for example, as part of an activity program or at special times, but not as continuous background music.

- People are given a great deal of privacy. Too much stimulation for the person with Alzheimer's disease is tiring and distressing. Therefore, it is essential there be provision for the individual to have plenty of privacy.

- Caregivers encourage residents to be active and participate in activities. People with dementia may require more encouragement and more individual attention to become involved.

- Personal grooming is evident. Caregivers oversee the personal grooming by encouraging individuals to perform as much of their own grooming as possible. Caregivers provide the grooming the individuals are unable to perform.

- Incontinence is managed in ways that preserve personal dignity. Incontinence is inevitable as the dementia progresses. Even though it may appear that people with dementia are not aware of their incontinence, it is imperative their dignity be maintained.

- Interactions among staff and people with Alzheimer's disease are pleasant and positive. Caregivers understand that people with Alzheimer's disease respond first to nonverbal then to verbal communication. Training for caregivers includes how to communicate and stresses the need for positive communication.

- The stress level of staff is low. Caregivers have chosen to work in the special care unit—they have been trained for the job and chosen to work with people with dementia. There are more staff per resident, which eases the work load. Caregivers in these units are given more freedom to act, along with more responsibility. Time is often provided for the staff to discuss their feelings and frustrations among their peers.

- Caregivers are very familiar with each person. The higher staff to resident ratio allows caregivers to spend more time with people living in the special care units.

- Therapeutic programs are functioning. Therapeutic programs (e.g., gardening) are designed especially to meet the needs of the people with dementia.

SAFETY ISSUES

If possible, the special care unit offers a safe outdoor exercise space where residents can walk outside, unattended and without danger of wandering off or hurting themselves. However, if the unit is carved out of an existing nursing home, safe outdoor exercise space may be limited or nonexistent. If such is the case, some environmental means may be used to keep the people with Alzheimer's disease from leaving the unit. Families may utilize these means at home, as well. Some precautionary steps to follow for creating a safe exercise space include the following:

- Develop indoor and outdoor areas where people can wander safely.

- Camouflage doors by painting them the same color as the wall.

- Place a large "NO!" or a red "STOP!" sign on doors.
- Place a full-length mirror on exit doors. They will cause some people to turn around when they see an image because they do not recognize themselves.
- Install an alarm system that sounds when the exit door is opened if the alarm has not been disengaged.

The overall benefits for both the caregivers and people with Alzheimer's disease are considerable. The satisfaction of the family is improved. And we can only believe the person with Alzheimer's disease is more comfortable.

Appendix A

Assessment Tools

Five tools frequently used to assess dementia or depression are presented in this appendix. All require a professional who is well-versed in taking medical histories by asking questions of the individual being assessed. Four tools rely on medical histories and one tool, Protocol for Evaluation of Dementia, uses medical history and the results of diagnostic tests. The latter tool would be completed by a physician or nurse.

The assessments requiring a medical history should be administered in a place that is familiar to the person being assessed, preferably in his or her home. In a familiar surrounding, the person will be less stressed. It is important the assessment be administered in a relaxed, unhurried manner. By administering the assessment in a familiar surrounding and in an unhurried fashion, it will be more accurate.

It may be necessary to administer an assessment more than once, especially if using one of the assessments that is relatively short and easier to administer, such as The Short Portable Mental Status Questionnaire (SPMSQ) and the VIRO Orientation Scale. For example, if a person is demonstrating difficulties with memory, the SPMSQ could be administered while at the same time checking for a medical cause for the memory problems. A few weeks later, if the symptoms persist, the same assessment should be administered again. This thoroughness will rule out single episodes of memory problems that may be caused by medication and physical problems.

Each completed assessment should be evaluated by a physician or nurse who is experienced in geriatrics and dementia. Following is a brief explanation of each of the tools:

- The Short Portable Mental Status Questionnaire requires the least amount of discernment on the part of the professional administering the assessment. Questions are phrased as they would be asked with space provided for responses. The responses should be written verbatim. If it is suspected a person is having memory problems, this is a good tool to use.

- The VIRO Orientation Scale requires the professional to formulate the questions, then record whether the answer is correct or not correct or within a certain number of years of the correct answer. This is also a good tool to use if it is suspected a person is having memory problems.

- The Geriatric Depression Scale can be used to evaluate if a person is depressed. This can be very helpful to use in conjunction with one of the assessments for dementia.

- The Folstein Mini-Mental Status Exam (MMSE) is a comprehensive evaluation of dementia and a more complex assessment to administer. It identifies the cognitive function being assessed with each question. It also provides instructions for the professional in delivering certain questions.

- The Protocol for Evaluation of Dementia requires information from diagnostic medical tests, such as blood tests and x-rays, in addition to a medical history. It may be necessary to obtain some of the information from the person's family or caregiver, depending on the person's mental condition. This tool looks for treatable causes of dementia. It provides an excellent summary of a person's physical and mental condition and may be placed in the person's chart.

THE SHORT PORTABLE
MENTAL STATUS QUESTIONNAIRE (SPMSQ)

Question	Response	Incorrect responses
1. What is the date, month, year?	_____	_____
2. What is the day of the week?	_____	_____
3. What is the name of this place?	_____	_____
4. What is your phone number (or address)?	_____	_____
5. How old are you?	_____	_____
6. When were you born?	_____	_____
7. Who is the current president?	_____	_____
8. Who was the president before him?	_____	_____
9. What was your mother's maiden name?	_____	_____
10. Can you count backward from 20 by 3s?	_____	_____

Scoring

0–2 errors: Normal mental functioning
3–4 errors: Mild cognitive impairment
5–7 errors: Moderate cognitive impairment
8 or more errors: Severe cognitive impairment

One more error is allowed in the scoring if the patient has had a grade school education or less. One less error is allowed if the patient has had education beyond the high school level.

From Pfeiffer, E. (1977). *The Short Portable Mental Status Questionnaire.* Tampa: Suncoast Gerontology Center, University of South Florida, Health Sciences Center; reprinted by permission.

VIRO ORIENTATION SCALE (*VIGOR, INTACTNESS, RELATIONSHIPS, ORIENTATION*)

Suitable for developing a spread of scores in very regressed patients. The respondent is awarded partial points for identifying the current year and his own age if he comes within ten years of the correct response. The orientation scale does not really tap dimensions reflecting more advanced cognitive abilities or even distant memory.

There is a .814 to .718 correlation with this test.

A perfect score (highest cognitive function measurable by this test) is 18.

			Score
1.	Knows age	Precisely	3
		Within 2 years	2
		Within 10 years	1
2.	Knows day of week	Yes	3
		No	0
3.	Knows month	Yes	3
		No	0
4.	Knows year	Precisely	3
		Within 2 years	2
		Within 10 years	1
		All else	0
5.	Knows name of community	Yes	3
		No	0
6.	Knows street	Yes	3
		No	0

From Reno, D.P. (1972). *Research, planning and action for the elderly.* New York: Plenum; reprinted by permission.

GERIATRIC DEPRESSION SCALE

1.	Are you basically satisfied with your life?	Yes	No
2.	Have you dropped many of your activities and interests?	Yes	No
3.	Do you feel that your life is empty?	Yes	No
4.	Do you often get bored?	Yes	No
5.	Are you hopeful about the future?	Yes	No
6.	Are you bothered by thoughts you can't get out of your head?	Yes	No
7.	Are you in good spirits most of the time?	Yes	No
8.	Are you afraid that something bad is going to happen to you?	Yes	No
9.	Do you feel happy most of the time?	Yes	No
10.	Do you often feel helpless?	Yes	No
11.	Do you often get restless and fidgety?	Yes	No
12.	Do you prefer to stay at home, rather than going out and doing new things?	Yes	No
13.	Do you frequently worry about the future?	Yes	No
14.	Do you feel you have more problems with memory than most?	Yes	No
15.	Do you think it is wonderful to be alive now?	Yes	No
16.	Do you often feel downhearted and blue?	Yes	No
17.	Do you feel pretty worthless the way you are now?	Yes	No
18.	Do you worry a lot about the past?	Yes	No
19.	Do you find life very exciting?	Yes	No
20.	Is it hard for you to get started on new projects?	Yes	No
21.	Do you feel full of energy?	Yes	No
22.	Do you feel that your situation is hopeless?	Yes	No
23.	Do you think that most people are better off than you are?	Yes	No
24.	Do you frequently get upset over little things?	Yes	No
25.	Do you frequently feel like crying?	Yes	No
26.	Do you have trouble concentrating?	Yes	No
27.	Do you enjoy getting up in the mornings?	Yes	No
28.	Do you prefer to avoid social gatherings?	Yes	No
29.	Is it easy for you to make decisions?	Yes	No
30.	Is your mind as clear as it used to be?	Yes	No

Scoring: One point for each answer.

1. no	6. yes	11. yes	16. yes	21. no	26. yes
2. yes	7. no	12. yes	17. yes	22. yes	27. no
3. yes	8. yes	13. yes	18. yes	23. yes	28. yes
4. yes	9. no	14. yes	19. no	24. yes	29. no
5. no	10. yes	15. no	20. yes	25. yes	30. no

Normal: 0–9
Mild depressives: 10–19
Severe depressives: 20–30

Source: Yesavage, Brink, Rose, Lum, Huang, Adey, & Leirer (1983).

THE FOLSTEIN
MINI-MENTAL STATUS EXAM (MMSE)

Cognitive function tested		Questions/tasks	Score
Orientation	1.	What is the year? Season? Date? Day? Month?	_____ (Maximum 5)
Orientation	2.	Where are we? State? County? Town? Hospital? Floor?	_____ (Maximum 5)
Registration	3.	Name three objects. The words are repeated until the patient learns all three. Examiner should allow 1 second to name each object to the patient, who is then asked to repeat the words immediately. Examiner should record the number of trials the patient needs to learn the three words. One point is given for each correct answer.	_____ (Maximum 3)
Attention & calculation	4.	Begin with the number 100 and subtract backward by 7s. Stop after five answers. If the patient does not enjoy arithmetic, ask him or her to spell "world" backward	_____ (Maximum 5)
Recall	5.	Repeat the three objects memorized above.	_____ (Maximum 3)
Language	6.	(Show the patient a pencil and watch.) Name each object.	_____ (Maximum 2)
Language	7.	Repeat the following: "No ifs, ands, or buts."	_____ (1)
Language	8.	(Ask the patient to follow a three-stage command.) Take this paper in your right hand, fold it in half, and put it on the floor.	_____ (Maximum 3)
Language	9.	Read and do the following instructions: "Close your eyes."	_____ (1)
Language	10.	Write a sentence.	_____ (1)
Language	11.	Copy this design.	_____ (1)
			_____ Total

Scoring

The lower the score, the greater the degree of impairment.
23 or less: Suggests cognitive impairment
30 points: Maximum

From Folstein, M.F., Folstein, S.E., & McHugh, P.R. (1975). Mini-Mental State: A practical guide for grading the cognitive state of patients for the clinician. *Journal of Psychiatric Research, 12,* 189–198; reprinted by permission.

PROTOCOL FOR EVALUATION OF DEMENTIA

HISTORY

Date of onset _____
Symptoms: Rapid _____   Gradual _____   Stepwise _____
Progression
    Uncertain _____
Drug history _____

History head trauma at time of onset   NO _____   YES _____
Depressive symptom   NO _____   YES _____
Hx CVA, TIA   NO _____   YES _____   Describe _____

PE

Localized neuro signs
Pathological reflexes   Absent _____   Present_____
Gait   Normal _____   Abnormal _____
Urinary incontinence   Absent _____   Present_____
Sensory exam   Normal _____   Abnormal _____
Depressive signs: Decreased appetite, sleep disturbance, helpless, hopeless, suicidal
    ideation
Hearing   Normal _____   Abnormal _____
Vision   Normal _____   Abnormal _____
Mental status exam MMSE (Folstein) _____   SPMSQ (Pfeiffer) _____

HACHINSKI ISCHEMIA SCORE

Characteristics	Point score
Abrupt onset	2
Stepwise deterioration	1
Somatic complaints	1
Emotional incontinence	1
History or presence of hypertension	1
History of strokes	2
Focal neurological symptoms	2
Focal neurological signs	2
Total Score: _____	

    Score of 4 or more suggests multi-infarct dementia

(continued)

From Pace, W. (1988). *Protocol for evaluation of dementia.* Unpublished manuscript; reprinted by permission of the author.

Protocol for evaluation of dementia　*(continued)*

DIAGNOSTIC STUDIES

	Normal	Abnormal
Blood		
CBC	_____	_____
Sedimentation rate	_____	_____
Glucose	_____	_____
BUN	_____	_____
Electrolytes	_____	_____
Calcium	_____	_____
Bilirubin	_____	_____
Free thyroxine index	_____	_____
TSH	_____	_____
VDRL	_____	_____
Vitamin B_{12}	_____	_____
Folate	_____	_____
Radiographic		
Chest x-ray	_____	_____
CT scan	_____	_____
Other		
Urinalysis	_____	_____
EEG	_____	_____
Lumbar puncture	_____	_____
Audiology	_____	_____

This may go into patient chart

Appendix B

Transparencies for Training Sessions

The supplemental material in this appendix can be removed from this book and made into transparencies to assist instructors during training sessions. The instructor should explain the transparencies by using material from the chapters and/or additional reading.

Guidelines for using and presenting overhead transparencies during training sessions appear in the Instructor's Guide. There also are tips for when to use the transparencies in the Instructor's Help sections after each Unit Quiz.

Instructions for making transparencies: Cut along the perforated marks at the edge of each page to remove from the book. Place transparency film in the paper tray of a photocopier. Place a page face down and copy. Please note that some photocopiers cannot be used to make transparencies. Older photocopiers tend to melt the transparency or jam. Transparency film usually can be purchased at office supply stores and will come in a package with instructions. Local copy centers also will make transparencies.

Unit 1

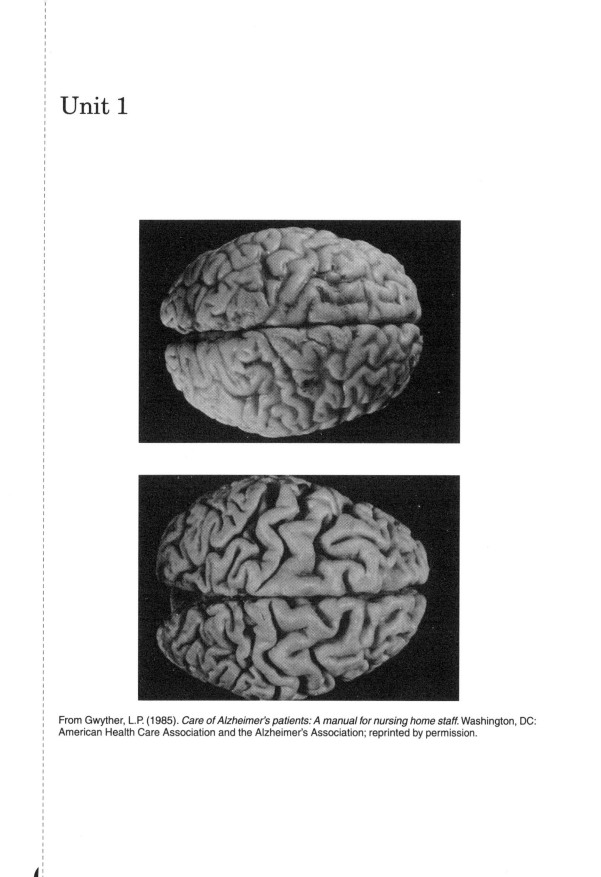

From Gwyther, L.P. (1985). *Care of Alzheimer's patients: A manual for nursing home staff.* Washington, DC: American Health Care Association and the Alzheimer's Association; reprinted by permission.

Unit 1

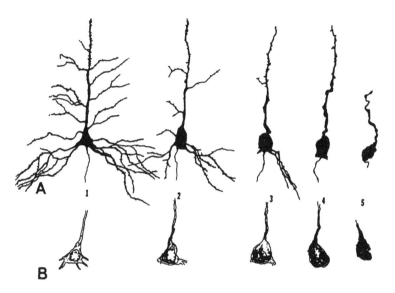

From Scheibel, M.E., Nandy, K., & Sherwin, L. (1977). *The aging brain and senile dementia.* New York: Plenum; reprinted by permission.

Unit 1

A Definition of Terms

Confusion   Reactions to environmental stimuli are inappropriate; person is bewildered or perplexed or unable to become oriented. Same as delirium if onset is sudden.

Delirium   A sudden onset mental status change that has an organic cause.

Dementia   A debilitating condition of the brain characterized by loss of memory, function, and personality.

Unit 1

Three Stages
of Alzheimer's Disease

First Stage
- Progressive forgetfulness
- Confusion about directions, decisions, and money management
- Loss of spontaneity and initiative
- Repetitive actions and statements
- Personality and judgment changes
- Disorientation of time and place

Three Stages
of Alzheimer's Disease

Second Stage
- Difficulty recognizing close friends and family
- Unable to retain new experiences
- Wandering
- Restlessness
- Occasional muscle twitching or jerking
- Difficulty organizing thoughts
- May be irritable, fidgety, or teary
- Becomes sloppy or confused about dressing
- May see or hear things that are not there
- Increased need for oral stimulation

Unit 1

Three Stages
of Alzheimer's Disease

Third Stage
- Loss of weight even with proper diet
- Unable to perform any daily care activities
- Communicates little or not at all
- Very irritable
- Loses ability to walk or sit up
- Sleeps more
- Death occurs

Unit 2

Verbal Communication

1. Dialogue
   - Use simple words.
   - Use simple sentences.
   - Give one command at a time.
   - Do not use pronouns.
   - Repeat a question or command.
   - Get a person's attention.

2. Style
   - Do not whisper.
   - Use face-to-face communication.
   - Speak slowly.
   - Speak in a quiet and calm voice.
   - Minimize environmental stimuli.

Unit 2

Nonverbal Communication

- Maintain eye contact.
- Touch the person gently.
- Exaggerate facial expressions, gestures, and body movements.
- Use a calm, gentle, and consistent approach.

Unit 3

Guidelines for Managing Personal Care

Toileting
- Mark the bathroom or bathroom door.
- Make sure the bathroom is accessible.
- Learn the person's urination and defecation schedule.
- Watch for agitation, restlessness, or pulling at clothing.
- Assist with clothing and positioning.
- Provide verbal cues.

Unit 3

Guidelines for Managing Personal Care

Bathing
- Adjust bathing schedule to the person's prior habits.
- Consider cultural background of the person.
- Avoid discussion about bathing.
- Stop if the person is severely agitated, angry, or frightened.
- Never leave the person unattended.
- Talk the person through each step.

Unit 3

Guidelines for Managing Personal Care

Dressing
- Decrease the number of choices.
- Lay out clothing items in their proper order.
- Replace buckles, buttons, and zippers.
- Lay out clothing that fastens in the back.

Unit 3

Guidelines for Managing Nutrition

Feeding
- Create as normal an eating situation as possible.
- Keep the eating experience positive.
- Offer a balanced diet.
- Be sure mouth care is performed at least twice a day.
- Consider prior eating habits.

Unit 4

Situation	Suggested Solution
Person refuses to take a bath.	Offer a shower. Try a different caregiver. Do not get angry. Leave resident alone. Offer again later.
Person is walking out the front door and going "home for lunch."	Say, "let's go together," walking in the same direction. Use the time to change the subject and slowly turn around.
Person repeats the same question over and over.	Ignore. He or she usually will stop asking.

Unit 6

Avoiding Burnout

1. Know what makes you angry or impatient.
2. Use mental imagery or visualization.
3. Use self-talk.
4. Evaluate the situation objectively.
5. Be flexible.
6. Take care of yourself physically, mentally, and spiritually.

Unit 6

Symptoms of Burnout Experienced by Caregivers

- Absenteeism
- Avoidance
- Chronic fatigue
- Depression
- Impatience
- Irritability
- Lack of enthusiasm
- Physical complaints

Appendix C

Suggested Readings

RESOURCES FOR PROFESSIONALS

The following is a list of articles, books, and audiotapes that offer supplemental information for each of the units. The asterisk (*) indicates resources that may also benefit family members.

Unit 1: Overview of Dementia

Bird, T.D., Nemens, E., & Kukull, W. (1993, September). Conjugal Alzheimer's disease: Is there an increased risk in offspring? *Annals of Neurology, 34*(3), 396–399.

*Blass, J., Ko, L., & Wisniewski, H. (1991). Pathology of Alzheimer's disease. *Psychiatric Clinics of North America, 14*(2), 397–441.

Burns, A., Jacoby, R., & Levy, R. (1991, January). Neurological signs in Alzheimer's disease. *Age Aging, 20*, 45–51.

*Exum, M., Phelps, B., Nabers, K., & Osborne, J. (1993). Sundown syndrome: Is it reflected in the use of PRN medications for nursing home residents? *Gerontologist, 33*(6), 756–761.

Farlow, M. (1993). Tacrine in the treatment of Alzheimer's disease. *Resident & Staff Physician, 39*(12), 39–47.

*Farlow, M., Gracon, S., Huskey, L., & Lewis, K. (1992). A controlled trial of tacrine in Alzheimer's disease. *Journal of the American Medical Association, 268*(18), 2523–2565.

Ghanbari, H. (1990). Biochemical assay of Alzheimer's disease—Associated proteins in human brain tissue. *Journal of the American Medical Association, 263*(21), 2907–2910.

*Hambdy, R., Turnbull, J., Clark, W., & Lancaster, M. (1994). *Alzheimer's disease—A handbook for caregivers* (2nd ed.). St. Louis: Mosby–Year Book.

Li, G., Silverman, J., & Mohs, R. (1991). Clinical genetic studies of Alzheimer's disease. *Psychiatric Clinics of North America, 14*(2), 267–284.

McDonald, W., & Nemeroff, C. (1991). Neurotransmitters and neuropeptides in Alzheimer's disease. *Psychiatric Clinics of North America, 14*(2), 421–434.

*McGowin, D. (1993). *Living in the labyrinth—A personal journey through the maze of Alzheimer's*. New York: Delacorte Press.

*Roth, M.E. (1993). Advances in Alzheimer's disease. *Journal of Family Practice, 37*(6), 593–607.

Scharnhorst, S. (1992, August). AIDS dementia complex in the elderly. *Nurse Practitioner*, pp. 37–39.

Staff. (1993, September). Tacrine for Alzheimer's disease. *Medical Letter*, *35*(905), 87–88.

Teri, L. (Producer). (1991). *Overview part I: Alzheimer's disease and related diseases* [Videotape]. Seattle: Alzheimer's Disease Research Center, University of Washington.

Teri, L. (Producer). (1991). *Overview part II: Delirium and depression* [Videotape]. Seattle: Alzheimer's Disease Research Center, University of Washington.

van Dujin, C., Tanja, T., & Haaxma, R. (1992). Head trauma and risk of Alzheimer's disease. *American Journal of Epidemiology*, *135*(7), 775–782.

Unit 2: Communication

Abrignani, C., & Messenger, B. (1991). *Alzheimer's disease: Activities that work*. La Grange, TX: M & H Publishing.

Beisgen, B. (1990). *Life-enhancing activities for mentally impaired elders*. New York: Springer.

*Bowlby, C. (1993). *Therapeutic activities with persons disabled by Alzheimer's disease and related disorders*. Rockville, MD: Aspen Publishers, Inc.

Clements, C.B. (1994). *The arts/fitness quality of life activities program: Creative ideas for working with older adults in group settings*. Baltimore: Health Professions Press.

Edwards, A. (1994). *When memory fails—Helping the Alzheimer's and dementia patient*. New York: Plenum.

*Feil, N. (1993). *The validation breakthrough—Simple techniques for communicating with people with "Alzheimer's-type dementia."* Baltimore: Health Professions Press.

*Hoffman, S., & Platt, C. (1991). *Comforting the confused*. New York: Springer.

Sheridan, C. (1991). *Reminiscence—Uncovering a lifetime of memories*. San Francisco: Elder Press.

Stevens, S. (1992). Differentiating the language disorder in dementia from dysphasia—The potential of a screening test. *European Journal of Disorders of Communication*, *27*(4), 278–288.

Teri, L. (Producer). (1991). *Managing aggressive behaviors: Anger, irritation, and catastrophic reactions* [Videotape]. Seattle: Alzheimer's Disease Research Center, University of Washington.

Teri, L. (Producer). (1991). *Managing psychotic behaviors: Language deficits* [Videotape]. Seattle: Alzheimer's Disease Research Center, University of Washington.

Teri, L., & Logsdon, L. (1991). Identifying pleasant activities for Alzheimer's disease patients: The pleasant events schedule. *Gerontologist*, *31*, 124–127.

Weingartner, H., Kawas, C., Rawlings, R., & Shapiro, M. (1993). Changes in semantic memory in early stage Alzheimer's disease patients. *Gerontologist*, *33*(5), 637–643.

Unit 3: Managing Personal Care and Nutrition

Brooks, J., Kraemer, H., Tank, E., & Yesavage, J. (1993). The methodology of studying decline in Alzheimer's disease. *Journal of American Geriatric Society*, *41*, 623–628.

Escott-Stump, S. (1992). *Nutrition and diagnosis related care* (3rd ed.). Washington, DC: Serif Press.

Green, C., Mohs, R., Schneidler, J., Aryan, M., & Davis, K. (1993). Functional decline in Alzheimer's disease: A longitudinal study. *Journal of American Geriatric Society, 41*, 654–661.

Hellen, C. (1994). *Alzheimer's disease—Activity focused care*. New York: Andover Medical Publishing.

*Robinson, A., Spencer, B., & White, L. (1991). *Understanding difficult behaviors: Practical suggestions for coping with Alzheimer's disease and related illnesses*. Ypsilanti: Geriatric Education Center of Michigan.

Skurla, E., Rogers, J., & Sunderland, T. (1988). Direct assessment of activities of daily living in Alzheimer's disease. *Journal of American Geriatric Society, 36*, 97–103.

Sloane, P., & Mathew, L. (1991). An assessment and care planning strategy for nursing home residents with dementia. *Gerontologist, 13*(1), 128–131.

Teri, L. (Producer). (1991). *Managing personal hygiene: Bathing and dressing* [Videotape]. Seattle: Alzheimer's Disease Research Center, University of Washington.

Unit 4: Managing Difficult Behaviors

*Ballard, E., & Poer, C. (1993). *Sexuality and the Alzheimer's patient*. Durham, NC: Duke Family Support Program, Duke University Medical Center.

*Braun, J., & Lipson, S. (Eds.). (1993). *Toward a restraint-free environment: Reducing the use of physical and chemical restraints in long-term and acute care settings*. Baltimore: Health Professions Press.

Cohen-Mansfield, J., Werner, P., & Marx, M. (1990). Screaming in the nursing home. *Journal of American Geriatric Society, 38*, 785–792.

Cooper, J., Mungas, D., & Weiler, P. (1990). Relation of cognitive status and abnormal behaviors in Alzheimer's disease. *Journal of American Geriatric Society, 38*, 867–870.

Dawson, P., & Reid, D.W. (1987). Behavioral dimensions of patients at risk of wandering. *Gerontologist, 27*, 104–207.

Deutsch, L., & Rovner, B. (1991). Agitation and other noncognitive abnormalities in Alzheimer's disease. *Psychiatric Clinics of North America, 14*(2), 341–349.

*Gwyther, L. (1985). *Care of Alzheimer's patients—A manual for nursing home staff*. Washington, DC: American Health Care Association and the Alzheimer's Association.

Robinson, A., Spencer, B., & White, L. (1991). *Understanding difficult behaviors—Some practical suggestions for coping with Alzheimer's disease and related illnesses*. Ypsilanti: Eastern Michigan University.

Szwabo, P., & Grossberg, G. (Eds.). (1992). *Problem behaviors in long-term care—Recognition, diagnosis, and treatment*. New York: Springer.

Teri, L. (Producer). (1991). *Managing difficult behaviors: Wandering and inappropriate sexual behaviors* [Videotape]. Seattle: Alzheimer's Disease Research Center, University of Washington.

Unit 5: Medications for Depression and Behavior Amelioration

Blair, D.T., & Dauner, A. (1992). Extrapyramidal symptoms are serious side-effects of antipsychotic and other drugs. *Nurse Practitioner Journal, 17*(11), 56–60.

*Farlow, M. (1991). A controlled trial of tacrine in Alzheimer's disease. *Journal of the American Medical Association, 268*(18), 2523–2527.

Handbook of psychotropic drugs. (1993). Springhouse, PA: Springhouse Corporation.

*Long, J.W., & Rybocki, J. (1994). *The essential guide to prescription drugs.* New York: Harper Collins.

Tune, L., Steele, C., & Cooper, T. (1991). Neuroleptic drugs in the management of behavioral symptoms of Alzheimer's disease. *Psychiatric Clinics of North America, 14*(2), 353–367.

Unit 6: Supporting the Caregivers—Staff and Families

*Anderson, K., Hobson, A., Steiner, P., & Rodel, B. (1992). Patients with dementia: Involving families to maximize nursing care. *Journal of Gerontological Nursing, 18*(7), 19–26.

Coughlin, P.B. (1993). *Facing Alzheimer's—Family caregivers speak.* New York: Ballantine.

*Gallienne, R., Moore, S., & Brennan, P. (1993). Alzheimer's caregivers: Psychosocial support via computer networks. *Journal of Gerontological Nursing, 19*(12), 15–23.

Harris, P.B. (1993). The misunderstood caregiver? A qualitative study of the male caregivers of Alzheimer's disease victims. *Gerontologist, 3*(4), 551–556.

Kiezer, J., & Fliss, L.C. (1991). Interview strategies to use in counseling families of demented patients. *Journal of Gerontology, 17*(1–2), 201–216.

*Lieberman, M., & Kramer, J. (1991). Factors affecting decisions to institutionalize demented elderly. *Gerontologist, 31*(3), 371–374.

Mullan, J. (1992). The bereaved caregiver: A prospective study of changes in well-being. *Gerontologist, 32*(5), 673–683.

Nick, S. (1992). Long-term care: Choices for geriatric residents. *Journal of Gerontological Nursing, 18*(7), 11–19.

Robinson, A., Spencer, B., & White, L. (1988). *Understanding difficult behaviors.* Ypsilanti: Geriatric Education Center of Michigan.

*Ronch, J. (1993). *Alzheimer's disease: A practical guide for families and other caregivers.* New York: Crossroad Publications.

Teri, L. (Producer). (1991). *Caregiver issues* [Videotape]. Seattle: Alzheimer's Disease Research Center, University of Washington.

Wallsten, S.M. (1993). Comparing patterns of stress in daily experiences of elderly caregivers and non-caregivers. *International Journal of Aging and Human Development, 37*(1), 55–68.

Wright, L. (1993). *Alzheimer's disease and marriage.* Newbury Park, CA: Sage Publications.

Unit 7: Special Care Units

Calkins, M. (1988). *Design for dementia: Planning environments for elderly and the confused.* Owings Mills, MD: National Health Publishers.

Christenson, M. (1990). *Aging in the designed environment.* New York: The Haworth Press.

Conrad, K., & Buttman, R. (1991). Characteristics of Alzheimer's versus non-Alzheimer's adult day care centers. *Research and Aging, 13*, 96–116.

Gold, D.T., Sloane, P., Mathew, L., Bledsoe, M., & Konanc, D. (1991). Special care units: A typology of care settings for memory impaired older adults. *Gerontologist, 31*, 467–475.

*Lawton, M.P. (1991). *Respite for caregivers of Alzheimer patients*. New York: Springer.

*Namazi, K., Rosner, T., & Calkins, M. (1989). Visual barriers to prevent ambulatory Alzheimer's patients from exiting through an emergency door. *Gerontologist, 29*(5), 699–702.

Peppard, N. (1991). *Special needs dementia units*. New York: Springer.

RESOURCES FOR FAMILIES

This reading list is not meant to be a complete bibliography. It contains selected readings that may be particularly helpful. Families also may benefit from some of the books and articles listed under "Resources for Professionals" that are marked with an asterisk (*).

References

These books address many of the issues family members commonly face in caring for a relative with a dementing illness. Practical advice for coping with the medical, legal, financial, and emotional aspects of care is provided.

American Association of Retired Persons. (1990). *Coping and caring: Living with Alzheimer's disease*. Washington, DC: Author.

Atlanta Alzheimer's Association. (1988). *Understanding and caring for the person with Alzheimer's disease: A practical guide*. Atlanta, GA: Author.

Carroll, D. (1989). *When your loved one has Alzheimer's: A caregiver's guide*. New York: Harper & Row.

Cohen, D., & Eisdorfer, C. (1986). *The loss of self*. New York: Norton.

Dippel, R., & Huston, J.T. (Eds.). (1991). *Caring for the Alzheimer's patient* (2nd ed.). Buffalo, NY: Prometheus.

Fish, S. (1990). *Alzheimer's: Caring for your loved one, caring for yourself*. Batavia, IL: Lion Publishing Co.

Mace, N., & Rabins, P. (1991). *The 36-hour day*. Baltimore: The Johns Hopkins University Press.

Powell, L. (1992). *Alzheimer's disease: A guide for families*. Menlo Park, CA: Addison-Wesley.

Diaries

The books included in this section have been written by families of people with Alzheimer's disease or by individuals with Alzheimer's disease. They describe the emotional turmoil faced when coping with the disease.

Ball, A.J. (1986). *Caring for an aging parent: Have I done all I can?* Buffalo, NY: Prometheus Books.

Bauer, C. (1987). *When I grow too old to dream: A journal on Alzheimer's disease*. New York: Vantage Press.

Davis, R. (1989). *My journey into Alzheimer's disease: A true story*. Wheaton, IL: Tyndale House.

Doernberg, M. (1989). *Stolen mind: The slow disappearance of Ray Doernberg*. Chapel Hill, NC: Algonquin Books of Chapel Hill.

Honel, R. (1988). *Journey with Grandpa: Our family's struggle with Alzheimer's disease*. Baltimore: The Johns Hopkins University Press.

Wirsig, W. (1990). *I love you, too!* New York: M. Evans and Company.

Institutional Care

The books listed below discuss considerations families need to think about when choosing a care facility for an aging relative.

Horne, J. (1989). *The nursing home handbook: A guide for families*. Washington, DC: American Association of Retired Persons.

Thompson, W. (1988). *Aging is a family affair: A guide to quality visiting, long term care facilities and you*. Toronto, Ontario, Canada: NC, Press Ltd.

Activities

These books discuss approaches in designing therapeutic activities for people with dementing illnesses. These activities can be done in the home, residential care settings, and adult day care settings. (Also see references for activities under Unit 2: Communication, in the Resources for Professionals section.)

Freeman, S. (1987). *Activities and approaches for Alzheimer's*. Knoxville, TN: The Whitfield Agency.

Sheridan, C. (1987). *Failure free activities for the Alzheimer's patient*. Oakland, CA: Cottage Books.

Children

These are illustrated stories for children 4–8 years old that describe what happens to a grandparent with Alzheimer's disease.

Guthrie, D. (1986). *Grandpa doesn't know it's me*. New York: Human Sciences Press.

Karkowsky, N. (1989). *Grandma's soup*. Rockville, MD: Kar-Ben Copies, Inc.

Kibbey, M. (1988). *My grammy*. MN: Carol Rhoda Books.

Noyes, L. (1982). *What's wrong with my grandma?* Falls Church: Northern Virginia Alzheimer's Association.

Teenagers

These books have been written for adolescents who want to learn more about Alzheimer's disease and the challenges that face both the person with Alzheimer's disease and the family as the disease progresses.

Frank, J. (1985). *The silent epidemic*. Minneapolis, MN: Lerner Publications Company.

Young, A. (1986). *What's wrong with Daddy?* Worthington, OH: Willowisp Press.

Newsletters

Alzheimer's Disease Newsletter
Alzheimer's Association (ADRDA)
919 North Michigan Ave., Suite 1000
Chicago, Illinois 60611-1676

Caregiving
Newsletter of Family Caregivers of the Aging
National Council on the Aging
600 Maryland Avenue, SW
West Wing 100
Washington, DC 20024

Parent Care: Resources to Assist Family Caregivers
Gerontology Center
316 Strong Hall
The University of Kansas
Lawrence, Kansas 66045
(913) 864-4130

Resource Centers

National Alzheimer's Association
919 North Michigan Ave., Suite 1000
Chicago, Illinois 60611-1676
(800) 272-3900

National Alzheimer's Disease Education and Referral (ADEAR) Center
Post Office Box 8250
Silver Spring, Maryland 20907-8250
(301) 495-3311

Appendix D

Answers to Unit Quizzes

UNIT 1: OVERVIEW OF DEMENTIA

1. a
2. a, b, d
3. True
4. False
5. c
6. b

UNIT 2: COMMUNICATION

1. False
2. False
3. False
4. c
5. c
6. b
7. b
8. False

UNIT 3: MANAGING PERSONAL CARE AND NUTRITION

1. a
2. c
3. True
4. False
5. b
6. Answers may include: Thicker liquids, moistened foods, serve liquids at room temperature, check mouth for stored food, give plenty of time between bites, gently stroke throat.

7. Answers may include: Warm room, well-lit bathroom, privacy, familiar caregivers.

8. c

9. laugh

UNIT 4: MANAGING DIFFICULT BEHAVIORS

1. Answers may include: Reassure person about where he or she is and why, do not confront or argue, speak in a calm voice, offer bathroom.

2. Answers may include: Decrease noise levels, remove triggers such as coat, camouflage doors, camouflage door knobs.

3. True

4. True

5. b

6. Speak gently

7. Frustration

8. True

9. True

UNIT 5: MEDICATIONS FOR DEPRESSION AND BEHAVIOR AMELIORATION

1. Answers may include: Constipation, dry mouth, orthostatic hypotension, urinary retention, glaucoma, blurred vision, paradoxical reactions, tardive dyskinesia, akathisia.

2. True

3. True

4. True

5. b

6. c

7. False

8. a

UNIT 6: SUPPORTING THE CAREGIVERS

1. True

2. Answers may include: Anger, helplessness, guilt, embarrassment

3. b
4. a
5. True
6. True
7. Answers may include: Giving information to family, being supportive, listening.
8. Answers may include: Past history and behavior management.

Index

Page numbers in italics denote figures; those followed by "t" denote tables.

Other important titles
from Health Professions Press . . .

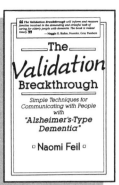

The Validation Breakthrough
Simple Techniques for Communicating with
People with "Alzheimer's-Type Dementia"

By **Naomi Feil, M.S.W.,** Validation Training Institute

*"With this technique . . . the confused person . . . [is] brought comfort and a sense of
resolution. . . . I heartily recommend this book to the long-term care industry."*
— **The Journal of Long-Term Care Administration**

"The many superbly presented vignettes bring the work from words to life."
— **Educational Gerontology**

In this bestselling book, internationally recognized expert Naomi Feil describes her simple but
effective approach for communicating with people with dementia. Based on decades of work with
older adults, Feil's techniques take just minutes a day and can be used by both family and professional caregivers to dramatically enhance the quality of their interactions with people at each stage
of dementia.

Fifteen poignant case studies illustrate how Validation is used to handle problem behaviors and
reduce the sense of anger and frustration in caregivers and clients. Used in over 7,000 facilities
around the world, Validation will transform the way caregivers work with people with dementia.

1993/352 pages/paperback/ISBN 1-878812-11-4/$22.00

—— **Yes!** Please send me the following books and videos:

____ copy(ies) of Feil: **The Validation Breakthrough**/Stock #114/$22.00

____ copy(ies) of Wylde: **A Careguide for the Confused Resident** (videotape and study manual)/
Stock #173/$120.00*

____ copy(ies) of Wylde: **Study Manual for A Careguide for the Confused Resident/**
Stock #181/$21.00 (3 manuals per packet)*

*Video and study manuals are not returnable.

____ Payment enclosed   ____ Visa   ____ Mastercard

Credit card # _____ Expiration date: _____
Signature _____
Name _____ Daytime telephone (____) _____
Address _____
City _____ State _____ Zip _____

Send orders to: Department A • Health Professions Press • Post Office Box 10624 • Baltimore, Maryland 21285-0624

A Careguide for the Confused Resident

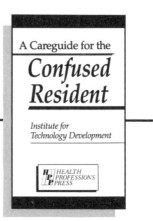

A Careguide for the
Confused
Resident

Institute for
Technology Development

*HP HEALTH
PROFESSIONS
PRESS*

Produced by the **Institute for Technology Development, Margaret A. Wylde, Ph.D.,** Project Director, from a project funded by the Retirement Research Foundation

This valuable training video prepares direct care providers to deal with confused behavior confidently and effectively. The video's seven thorough, clearly explained units take viewers step-by-step as nursing home staff learn to respond to various types of confusion in residents. Viewers will learn how to:

- *recognize when a resident is confused*
- *determine what factors are triggering the confusion*
- *set specific goals for desired behavior changes*
- *encourage new behavior patterns by rewarding positive changes*

Included in the price of the video is an extensive study manual that helps viewers retain what they learn by identifying learning objectives and key points of each unit shown in the video. Ideal for training in long-term care facilities, technical and vocational schools, and community colleges, this cost-effective training video can be used again and again to teach staff and students how to deal with confused behavior.

75 minutes/color/½″ VHS videocassette format/ISBN 1-878812-17-3/$120.00

Study Manual for
A Careguide for the Confused Resident

Available in packets of three, the **Study Manual for A Careguide for the Confused Resident** includes samples of completed forms, blank forms for staff or students to fill in, and questions (and their answers) to guide users through the process of developing a care plan. This convenient manual is the *only* text that staff or students need to get the full benefit of this video training program.

1994/60 pages each/7 × 10/saddle-stitched/ISBN 1-878812-18-1/$21.00

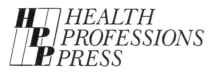

HP HEALTH PROFESSIONS PRESS

Post Office Box 10624 • Baltimore, MD 21285